DOCTORS
DISSECTED

DOCTORS DISSECTED

Jane Haynes & Martin Scurr

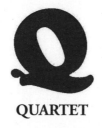

QUARTET

First published in 2015 by Quartet Books Limited
A member of the Namara Group
27 Goodge Street, London W1T 2LD
Copyright © Jane Haynes and Martin Scurr 2015
The right of Jane Haynes and Martin Scurr to be identified
as the authors of this work has been asserted
by them in accordance with the
Copyright, Designs and Patents Act, 1988
All rights reserved.
No part of this book may be reproduced in
any form or by any means without prior
written permission from the publisher
A catalogue record for this book
is available from the British Library
ISBN 978 0 7043 7375 4
Typeset by Josh Bryson
Printed and bound in Great Britain by
T J International Ltd, Padstow, Cornwall

2

For Blue-Ey'd Belle and Little Thea

CONTENTS

It is illness that makes us recognize that we do not live in isolation but are chained to a being from a different realm, worlds apart from us, with no knowledge of us and by whom it is impossible to make ourselves understood: our body.

Marcel Proust

INTRODUCTION

You're on earth. There's no cure for that.

Samuel Beckett

This is a storybook about medicine, body, mind, doctors and caprices of human nature written by an experienced doctor in his sixties (Martin Scurr), who has seen every untidy vagary of disease, and a psychotherapist of similar age (Jane Haynes), who has listened to personal narratives that rival the visceral emotions of *King Lear*. Doctors at their most profound are mercurial messengers between life and death. At a more comedic level doctors, who must suffer our jiggling body parts, are also behind their white masks vulnerable and sometimes flawed men and women struggling to make sense of their existence. They are the only people other than our lovers to whom we (if unwillingly) grant voluntary access to our bodies and their orifices. The degree of such intimacy is emphasized by the concern of all medical ethics which promises that we will not be taken advantage of should we fall ill and become infantilized. Hippocrates wrote, 'First do no harm.'*

Our intentions are fourfold: first we wish to explore the ways in which the figure of the twentieth century General Practitioner, trained to have a holistic and humanistic approach to his patients' health, often from birth to death, have been eroded. A revolution has occurred in the practice of general medicine in the UK, which has been effected through changes in successive government policies and the needs of a changing demography.

Secondly, we consider whether the idea of a family doctor, who was familiar with the names and medical *histories* of patients, has become a casualty of the NHS and a loss to the vocation of

---

* This injunction does not as is commonly assumed appear in the Hippocratic Oath, but in his later writings about the control of epidemics.

medicine. The increasing popularity of alternative and holistic medicines, which are more affordable than private medicine, is another indication that the public are disillusioned with the utility of their medical care and are seeking to complement it. More and more people are driven to compensate for the absence of time, the personal touch, or bedside manner, by seeking out a substitute in the form of a complementary practitioner who *remembers* them from one consultation to the next.

Thirdly, we will steal behind the mask, or professional persona, of the doctor to discover how the privileges, challenges and overbearing responsibilities of vocation impact upon private life. To these ends, in her role as psychotherapist, Jane has attempted an autopsy on Martin's professional, and where the two inevitably merge, his personal life; in other words, his existence. We will discover how the medical profession has changed over 40 years primarily through a series of interviews with Martin who qualified in 1973, illumined by memoir, and later on with his son Cosmo, who is currently in postgraduate training to become a consultant in Anaesthetics. The accounts of Cosmo's enthusiasm and passion for his vocation will allow the authors to avoid the pitfalls of a shared nostalgia in which the past can present itself as a golden age. Cosmo's medical school training at Imperial College, London has been different from his father's and whether it is improvement, impoverishment, or just different the reader must decide.

Last, but perhaps most important of all, we want to penetrate beyond the political issues into the heartlands of people who are drawn to a life in medicine; to explore through narrative what it means to choose a profession in which the practitioner is constantly being faced with lonely decisions that are often equivalent to life and death. To these ends we shall also interview other GPs both NHS and private, both young and retired, about their lives and masked selves. Our intention is not to provide quantitative research into the career structures of our contributors' lives, but to explore the existential and emotional phenomena of choosing a career in medicine.

It is also clear from our interviewees that candidates for training come primarily although by no means exclusively from middle class families. Regardless of the familial and cultural origins of our contributors the choice of a medical career has rewarded all of them with financial, if not emotional security and a privileged position in society of authority and respect. The rewards and privileges of becoming a GP, whether in London, or Glasgow, whether driven by vocation or ambition, are undisputable and substantial, whereas the affluence or deprivation of their patients' lives will vary hugely according to geography and to their choice of employment. Salaried NHS GPs, who are part of a 'clinical commissioning group', can earn between £54,319 to £81,969 dependent on, among other factors, length of service and experience, while practice partners' earnings can reach £160,000. The same is not true of hospital doctors where even a senior specialist registrar will still only be earning in the region of £47,000 and the most senior full-time NHS consultant physician, or surgeon at the top the ladder is unlikely to earn more than £130,000, with the average being half that amount. As a point in comparison the *Guardian* stated: 'David Cameron and Ed Miliband will face embarrassment this week when it is announced that MPs will be paid an annual salary of £74,000 from 2015 despite their calls for "cheaper politics".'

Medicine is not just a job, a paid profession. Being a doctor means to become a member of a profession which historically has been put on a pedestal and is seen to be somehow different: respected, and even honoured, but also quickly reviled whenever it is found to be wanting. Ideally, its skill set demands a challenging combination of the objectivity of scientific professionalism with human warmth and sympathy which is difficult to predict in an 18-year-old applicant. The days of medical fathers proudly introducing their children to the deans of medical schools, offering them up for interview on the grounds that they show promise, play for a school's rugby team, or sing in the choir fortunately have come to an end but there is evidence that we still do not know how to select, out of the young people completing their secondary schooling, the best and most suitable candidates to train for a medical career.

Politically directed changes are annually taking place within the medical profession, which impact on the different ways that medical faculties are constructed and on the priorities of a medical training. Change is healthy and inevitable and it is also the backbone of science but there is increasing suspicion among the medical fraternity that such modifications are not always in either the best interest of patients, or the practice of medicine. These changes are best summed up in Dr Peter Holden's radio commentary on his official report on the 7/7 terrorist attacks. A bus was blown up outside of the British Medical Association headquarters where Holden, a specialist in trauma control, was by co-incidence attending a meeting.

One of the most amazing things that went on in the courtyard of the BMC on 7/7 was the general level of medical competence. One of my colleagues who I knew had not managed a seriously injured casualty for years reacted as though he had done it yesterday. I watched him put in an intravenous cannula which he had not done for 20 years. I'm in my mid fifties and I had a fairly broad medical training and this incident has caused me to reflect on what is happened to medical training today. When I trained we were allowed to pick and mix our jobs at junior doctor level before pitching in to any specialization. It was then regarded as important that we had had a broad training which pitched us into experiences of the generalities of medicine before we had to decide which speciality we wanted to go into. It's not like that today and God forbid we should have an emergency in 2020 or 2025 I worry whether the doctors there would still have the breadth of training necessary to cope with the state of emergency. Already we are seeing, in some areas of medicine, over specialization when young doctors still need to be educated to have a breadth of knowledge. There is nothing wrong with specialization except today's student doctors have to make their minds up so very quickly and often they are even required to make the decision the moment they qualify and that is crazy. My anxiety is that we are no longer training the students to be a bunch of professionals but that they are being trained for a job in the health service with all that implies. There is an increasing risk that medical students are now being trained to fill a slot rather than to become a doctor.

We will introduce ourselves more fully.

As a psychotherapist I also convene professional development groups for doctors and consultant psychiatrists. The focus of the group is not on doctors discussing, or reflecting on their interactions with, or anxieties about their patients. Rather, the focus is on the group's own conflicting emotions and concealed fears relating to both authority and helplessness, science and magical thinking, or the greed, ambition and altruism that often co-exist inside the doctor's psyche. An act of serendipity brought about my introduction to Martin whose reputation as a distinguished Physician and Fellow of the Royal College of Physicians and the Royal College of General Practitioners, travels before him. It is not uncommon for his patients to travel across counties, or even countries for a diagnostic consultation.

Martin comes from a family of doctors: his father was a doctor; two of his siblings are doctors, as are several first cousins, and as mentioned earlier, his son Cosmo recently qualified as a doctor. Martin is an example of a doctor whose passionate devotion to medicine and lifetime study of its advanced sciences is apparent to his colleagues and to his patients. I have the impression of him always in an enthusiastic hurry to arrive, vibrating with energy but unlike the White Rabbit, rarely visibly impatient, or clock-watching as he races between one patient's needs and the next. The time of day, night, or week makes no difference to his willingness to answer his mobile, or to visit a patient at home. His vocational energy has been sustained and accompanied by a private life equally rich in its variety and emotional experiences. He married only once but has children from three partners.

I wanted to be a doctor myself but my education did not include entering a science laboratory so that became an unlikely possibility. Instead in my late teens, while I was waiting for acting jobs, I found myself working as a temporary medical secretary. I must have cost the Middlesex Hospital a fortune through my atrocious typing at a time when carbon paper with Tipp-ex was still employed and I had to provide six copies of every correspondence. I would leave hospital each evening, my handbag bulging with headed vellum paper, on which I had made multiple mistakes. One unforgettable day the secretarial agency called and shipped me off to Morbid Anatomy at Bart's Hospital. Naïve, I had no idea where, as the lift ascended to the rooftop, I was to arrive. It became evident that I was in unfamiliar and chilly surroundings where everyone looked messy and there was an obtrusive, damp smell. It was not until I was asked to take dictation that I discovered I was in the anteroom of the morgue. I found myself transcribing data about the relentless abnormalities of one newborn infant. My horror at the pitiless and scientific description of the suffering of a brief life chilled me

INTRODUCTION

to the core and fuelled me with nightmare terrors about my own fertility. Without explanation, I returned to the lift and left the building; but the dreams about that small and nameless child, and the smoking incinerator into which I knew his body had been dispatched have pursued me.

Since that early experience in the Department of Morbid Anatomy I have remained intrigued to know why anyone would choose to spend their life absorbing pain and suffering. Poets and musicians, novelists and painters, perhaps all creative artists are inspired by the emotional life and the intensity of feelings like love, jealousy, and nostalgia, but there is no affliction of the soul that can equal the body in pain. Pain, disease and the battle against mortality are the daily bread and butter of a doctor's life. Doctors, unlike any other professional status other than teachers, inevitably play a critical part in everybody's life. The Emperor Hadrian observed during his mortal illness that it was impossible even for an emperor to remain an emperor when he stood naked in front of his physician. Nobody can escape the doctor.

Death is also associated with the magic of rebirth and the doctor today is still depicted with his symbolic magic wand, the snake rod of Asclepius the Greek god of medicine. When we visit the antiseptic and enclosed consultation space beneath those hygienic, secular and plastic surfaces, we are also calling upon the doctor's cultural links, which go back to ancient times with their sacred energies and prescriptive spells and potions, to renew life. Doctors witness our beginnings and our endings, we cannot be buried without their signature, and probably they will turn out to be the messengers of our mortality. Doctors receive our childlike transferences of gratitude, disappointment and even rage. Children expect their doctor to make them better and to stop them hurting. Adults still hold on to the myth that the doctor will magically, even if not always scientifically, be able to save life. Yet, doctors are often, like their patients, afraid of illness because they know better than anybody the limits and potential ugly consequences of the side effects of medicine and science on our bodies and our mortality.

Doctors feature powerfully in universal histories and in literature across civilizations and generations, illustrating the strength of our fascination with their attributed powers. Doctors of one kind or another have been portrayed in many ways over the centuries through fiction, drama and more recently television. Chaucer and Shakespeare were both fascinated by medicine's magical and scientific properties but whereas King Lear's doctor embodied wisdom, Macbeth's doctor was a coward. Whether good or evil, stories and dramas about medical practitioners have always grabbed the attention of the reader. Marlowe's *Dr Faustus*, both polymath and physician, was not satisfied with the limits of his mortal knowledge and entered into a pact with the Devil. Ian Fleming's *Dr No* battled James Bond for world domination. There is Dr Van Helsing, the doc in Bram Stoker's *Dracula*, or Mary Shelley's *Frankenstein*, and Stevenson's Dr Jekyll, not to exclude Camus' plague doctor Dr Rieux. Tennyson ('In the Children's Hospital') provides us with a nightmare of Shipman-like proportions:

> **OUR** doctor had call'd in another, I never had seen him before,
> But he sent a chill to my heart when I saw him come in at the door,
> Fresh from the surgery-schools of France and of other lands—
> Harsh red hair, big voice, big chest, big merciless hands!
> Wonderful cures he had done, O, yes, but they said too of him
> He was happier using the knife than in trying to save the limb,
> And that I can well believe, for he look'd so coarse and so red,
> I could think he was one of those who would break their jests on
> the dead.

8

INTRODUCTION

Many other authors have used doctors as their main character in order to provide us with insight into the way doctors operate: from H. G. Wells' *The Island of Dr Moreau* to the classic *Doctor Zhivago*, by Boris Pasternak. A. J. Cronin, himself a doctor, wrote the influential *The Citadel* and it was out of this novella that the television series, *Dr Finlay's Casebook* was devised. Bulgakov, perhaps the most subversive of Communist writers was also a doctor whose first book was an account of his experiences in the Russian rural and isolated province of Smolensk. Most recently Sarah Waters and Ian McEwan have fastened on to the power of doctors to fascinate their readers, while Martin himself is the medical advisor on *Doc Martin*.

Little surprise then that two of the 19th century's greatest European novels explore the moral contradictions apparent both in our own tangled relationships with doctors, and those of doctors themselves. Through *Madame Bovary*, Flaubert explored his maxim that all doctors were materialists and that 'you can't probe for faith with a scalpel' while George Eliot's Dr Lydgate in *Middlemarch* wrestles similarly:

> Many of us looking back through life would say that the kindest man we have ever known has been a medical man, or perhaps the surgeon whose fine tact, directed by deeply informed perception, has come to our need with a more sublime beneficence than that of miracle workers. Some of the twice-blessed mercy was always with Lydgate in his work at the Hospital or in private houses, serving better than any opiate to quiet and sustain him under his anxieties and his sense of mental degeneracy.

In both of these novels, as in most of the others listed above, the doctor is a familiar both in the social life of the community and in his patients' homes, where his presence brings an immediate if occasionally misplaced sense of relief and trust in his authority and wisdom. Unlike today, where as we shall hear from Cosmo, 'out of hours' medicine is in danger of being confused with 'emergency medicine', those rural doctors would think little of travelling across difficult or even dangerous terrains to attend their patients at home.

While my children were growing up the welcome arrival of our family doctor to diagnose an acute ear infection late at night was not uncommon. I remember our small son clambering the nursery curtains, pleading for his 'friend' our doctor to arrive, driven by the relentless pain in his ears. I can also remember our doctor – a dapper man by day – sitting past midnight on our son's bunk bed and delicately checking his throat and ears. Dr Smith, who spent his days in pinstripes, wafted *Eau Sauvage* and stole wet-lipped kisses from some of his lady patients – but only at his door where he 'courteously' stood sentinel to bid them goodbye – had arrived in jeans and an open neck, if crisp and wife-ironed, striped shirt. How young he looked: I had always thought of him as old, but what then took me by surprise, as he knelt down by the bunk, was a gold chain and the flash of a most unlikely over-sized and sparkling medallion recessed into his rowdy chest. At this clash of aesthetic, his gravitas morphed and I realised that he was another 'ordinary' man who concealed behind his day-consulting-patina all sorts of quirks, vanities and clues to another life beyond the limited one to which I had access. Long retired and dead now, I still have an image of him sitting pinstripe elegant behind his mahogany desk, fountain pen poised, with which he entered in long hand, those medical tidings – both benign and malignant – of patient mortalities into a leather bound manuscript.

Now it is becoming rare for doctors ever to enter their patients' homes, or even to remember their names before they glance towards their computers. Some futurist physicists like Michio Kaku are predicting that before the end of the century microsurgery will be conducted remotely over the Internet. Regardless of predictions from the futurist physicists there needs to be something sacred about our health, because health is the opposite to disease and thus a visit to the doctor will subliminally remind us of our mortality and our prospective death.

How rarely are our GPs now available to be summoned in those lonely hours of the early morning, which are most disposed to seeing the dying depart. While we may have to accept that along with the population explosion there are many ideals of leisured medical consultation that belong to the past there is something awful happening when patients cannot expect to be remembered, or attended to, except by a stranger in their hours of greatest need and terror. During the swine 'flu debacle of 2009, I was told by a family member, who is a specialist in infectious disease control, that it was not uncommon to witness anxious parents arriving at a medical centre in Lambeth only to be instructed to remain in their car until a doctor in full protective environmental suiting and mask, emerged to thrust a do it yourself swab kit through the car window. What will happen, as Dr Holden has also asked, to the doctor and patient relationship when a major environmental infectious disaster strikes at the heart of society? Between one day and the next, and usually without warning a trickster virus can descend, or a stroke paralyze us. Too easily we are able to eradicate the facts of the 1918 'flu epidemic, which infected 500 million people across the world and killed between 50 and 100 million of them.

When something goes wrong with our body, or our children's bodies, we are immediately vulnerable and liable, if not forced, to abandon our autonomy and place ourselves in what may be an uncomfortable, or even a hostile stranger's hand. Depending on how ill or vulnerable we feel, we may, or may not fear that we are falling apart. Illness creates disorder: 'Things fall apart/The centre cannot hold/Mere anarchy is loosed upon the world.' We need only to substitute 'upon the body' for Yeats' lines to serve as a description for what can happen when we are suddenly 'taken' acutely ill. (Note the sense of fateful intervention in the metaphoric use of the verb, 'taken'.) Many connections are severed and taken away as illness isolates us from the familiar routines of our lives and renders us most vulnerable.

A friend of mine was having her first consultation with an oncologist and she was anxious to try and make sense of a sequence of events, which had overnight changed her identity from that of a healthy person into a woman with a terminal disease. Her narrative was cut short by the consultant, 'I am not interested in your life, I am interested in your symptoms.' What is more important to a patient than their life, and particularly if there is a terminal threat? Martin's student colleague at the Westminster Hospital dissecting tables, who is now Professor of Complementary Medicine and Research at the University of Southampton, George Lewith suggests:

> There's a lot about the human spirit which comes through in complementary medicine; I think it's a metaphor for lots of things we are missing in conventional medicine rather than necessarily as proven valid therapies in themselves and there's still a great deal of meaning in the process of complementary medicine which we need to understand. We need to remember and cherish the human need for spirituality: where there is equality of dialogue, where touch, whether touching the body or spirit is a part of the therapy which is also critical to health and recovery and I think there's a big element of modern medicine where all this is denied or undervalued.

INTRODUCTION

Lewith's comments return us to the debate about the importance of a doctor's bedside manner, or 'healing touch'. Something different can happen to our body when we are welcomed into the consulting room not by a stranger but by a doctor with whom we may have established a relationship, or have been attended by in our own beds. The doctor by remembering us is able at a symbolic and unspoken level to use his medical skills to re-member us. It is only over 'time' that a doctor is best able to care for, and to understand what is best for his patient, and to win their trust in his assessment. Pain is one of the most subjective of human experiences and it is with continuity of care that a doctor will be better able to 'measure' pain and suffering.

1
MARTIN ASKS...

January 2010

Do the children of doctors study medicine because of an innate understanding of what is involved, which has been imbued during a childhood of exposure? I find this is hard to believe; the life of a pathologist is so different from the life of a GP and so different again from the world of an anaesthetist. Yet, those children will from an early age become aware that they have a parent who is a doctor in the most prominent position among the healing professions. Could it be that what fuels their early determination to become a doctor is the result of an involuntary access to the mysterious and powerful knowledge that their parent holds, or their observations that being a doctor is seen to involve a special, even privileged position in our society? That respect and honour has a timeless history: long before Hippocrates became established in ancient Greece as the father of modern medicine, the Egyptians already had the experience of centuries of organized and specialized medical care; rulers of distant empires would ask Pharaohs to send them their best physicians to provide advice. An ancient scroll records a correspondence between Egypt and the Anatolian kingdom of Hatti during the reign of Rameses II, when Hattusili III appealed to Rameses to send him an expert to treat his sterile sister Matananzi. The Pharaoh agreed:

> Now see here as for Matananzi my brother's sister (I) the king your brother knows her...50, is she? She is 60 for sure...no one can produce medicine for her to have children. But of course if the Sun God (of Egypt) and the Storm God (of Hatti) should will it...but I will send an able physician and a good magician and they can prepare some birth drugs for her...(anyway).

MARTIN ASKS…

There seems to be a social attachment to the idea that those of us who practise medicine, through our practical associations with life and death, are beings apart, are different in some way, society inevitably taking note of an acknowledged special status, which has been intrinsic to many civilized and developed societies. The doctor makes, or perhaps the idea of such an act is now an anachronism, certain sacrifices in his life such as *his commitment to the well-being of his patient being as great, or greater than commitment to his own life*. In return for their ancient oath, society has honoured doctors with a degree of status and respect but one which is only retained when diligence and care continue to be evident. This sense of vocation, if not always devotion, was the case with the Egyptians, the Greeks, the Romans, and evolved along similar lines in Europe after the Dark Ages. Even today, for many parents there seems to be a special pride in having a child who declares: 'I want to be a doctor when I grow up.'

Something happened to me the other day that made me realize that I might even need the help of a psychotherapist! I found myself advising a young patient of mine, whom I have looked after since birth against applying to medical school. This intervention signified a 180-degree turnaround from the position I have held for the last 40 years since qualifying myself. What was happening that provoked this change from being devoted to the idea of a career in medicine to doing all I could to persuade a young idealist to reconsider his plans and ambitions? Without doubt, I must start to examine my conscience and the weight of a disillusion so recent that it even precedes my son Cosmo's graduation last year as a doctor. What is it about my profession that has caused me – in an uncharacteristic and impetuous manner – to dissuade an enthusiastic and talented individual from following a vocation, which since I was hardly out of short trousers, has provided me with almost lifelong pleasure?

DOCTORS DISSECTED

Cosmo, now a junior hospital doctor, was frequently and perhaps irritatingly asked in childhood if he hoped to follow in my footsteps. I recall his reply on one occasion, at around the age of eight: 'I couldn't bear to miss my breakfast.' Even when I did manage to get home to supper I was often busy with multiple telephone calls out of hours and responding to my pager which often produced two or three house visits each night and sometimes up to 20 home visits over a weekend. Cosmo's enduring experience of my fractured presence was seeing me leave meals early, or waiting in the car with his mother and brother as we travelled home from a family occasion elsewhere while I had to visit a patient at their home, or in hospital, en route, which is still something that is part of my daily schedule.

Cosmo's mother – a prominent professional in the film industry – was magnificent and tolerant in her approach to those intrusions into our family life. My wife was respectful, supportive, and patient with my activities and my adherence to various commitments, although she used occasionally to roll her eyes and talk about 'the awesome responsibility of the job'. She had her own critical health issues, having been found with her twin sister to have rickets at the age of seven: their legs were bowing due to the softening of bone caused by calcium abnormalities which were the consequence of a previously unknown kidney disease. Hers was not the traditional cause of rickets, which is a vitamin D deficiency caused by poor diet and lack of sunshine, but was renal osteodystrophy, where kidney malfunction affects the bones. The investigations for this mysterious condition were carried out at the nationally famous Hospital for Sick Children, Great Ormond Street, by the consultant responsible for their care, Sir Wilfred Sheldon, along with his senior registrar, Joe Luder, and their condition came to be known as the Sheldon-Luder syndrome. The disease was subsequently found to be due to an autosomal dominant gene, and along with the examination of the family tree came the realization that their father was also affected. It turned out that he died of septicaemia, after a kidney transplant at the age of 46 in 1976; looking further back, at least one other case in earlier generations was identified.

In this disease the kidney function ultimately fails in early middle age and my wife received a transplant from myself when we were both 42 which became an early example of a live but unrelated kidney donation kidney failure. My wife lost my kidney on the sixth post-operative day, which was due to a surgical complication when there was a thrombosis of her renal vein. By the time that this disaster happened we had discovered that both of our sons had the same diagnosis. They both grew up witnessing their mother struggling bravely with dialysis for 12 years before she was ultimately able to receive a second transplant when in her mid fifties from a distant cousin. The boys know, even as I write this, that they have the prospect of renal failure and transplantation ahead of them. At every level we were a medical household and there was a sense that father will look after everything and are we not fortunate to have the privilege of this in-house knowledge. Maybe, that sense of a fast track to anything that might ever be needed was seen by the family as one of the perks of having a father in the medical profession – some small consolation for the fact that he was so rarely home – 'When it is our turn he will be there for us.' At least that was the sense that I felt, loud and clear.

Towards the end of Cosmo's school days we determined to send him on sixth form work experience to both a magic circle law firm, a city investment banker and an architect's office. He had already spent much time during his school holiday working part-time as a technician on film sets, as an assistant clapper-loader, or focus puller. Nothing we did seemed to deter him from what had now become his ambition to become a doctor. After he graduated from school with distinctions in mathematics, chemistry and biology, core subjects for the future study of medicine he turned his back on the city and media and went to work as a porter in the same hospital where he was later to undertake a medical training. He quickly graduated to becoming a secretary in the radiology department. Afterwards, he spent many months in Ghana working in a similar position in a hospital, until he had been assured of his place at Imperial College Medical School in London. Strange, our parental ambivalence, as we had both had no doubt that we wanted to call him Cosmo, who is a patron saint of medicine. There was St Cosmo and St Damian who were Arabian twins born in the third century AD. Their most famous miraculous exploit was the grafting of a leg from a recently deceased Ethiopian to replace their patient's ulcerated leg, which became the subject of many paintings and illuminations. There is a painting by Fra Angelico of a noble man who is having a miraculous leg transplant by the brothers from a dead Negro. As a result of this seemingly miraculous surgery they became the patron saints of doctors and transplant surgeons.

Sometimes, I still wonder why Cosmo did not fall for the glitz and technology of filmmaking. Why, when my own exposure to that tantalizing world had already screwed my head on very firmly and I also knew about the inevitable boredom and long hours of film shoots? In fact an exposure to media came early in my career through having high profile individuals as patients and seeing firsthand the penalties that they sometimes paid for their fame and fortune in terms of loss of privacy, loss of perspective. Then, there are the private terrors and insecurities, which successful personas belie, but that can shadow entire lives, despite their public success and leave them susceptible to anxiety, stress related illness, depressions and even tragic suicides. Later, there were often occasions when I was invited to appear on current affairs and other minor TV and radio programmes, which reinforced my cautious cynicism about the delights of five minutes of fame. I have continued throughout my career to act as medical consultant on both feature films and television projects. Never, not even for a moment, did I ever feel that a career in the media, or politics, could be more interesting and fulfilling than my work in medicine, and yet I continued to be anxious about Cosmo following in my footsteps. There are, and have been regrets – more of that later – but then which of us, deep down is not aware that the grass in the next field always seems so much greener?

Now, I have a new fear: that medical training and commitment is changing as it becomes dictated to by the ever increasing bureaucratic needs of the National Health Service, and the irrevocable migration of commitment from a vocation, to the performance of a function which has become more like a technical job, curtailed by the 48-hour European working time directive, which I see will inevitably damage the emotional relationship that doctors have with both their subject and their patients. I recently reviewed a sickening book on patient care in the NHS that may have contributed to my volte-face with my young patient in which Michael Mandelstam, a consultant to the NHS, reveals the extremes of current patient neglect and suffering: *How We Treat the Sick: Neglect and Abuse in Our Health Services*.

This still would not however explain my earlier ambivalence about Cosmo's decision when the practice of medicine by the individuals of my own extended family does seem to have become inevitable. My sister and one brother also graduated from London medical schools. My cousin is a consultant vascular surgeon, one of his sons is also a vascular surgeon, and one daughter is a paediatrician, while another of his daughters has just graduated and like Cosmo is now a junior hospital doctor. My father was the first member in our family to enter the medical profession, when he received his medical degree in 1942. His younger brother died of cancer at the age of 21 while at medical school some years later. Their father and his brother were both opticians and men who had had scientific backgrounds and an intellectual professional training. The older, my grandfather, had initially trained as a pharmacist but he then became an optician, and it seems he then trained his brother to become an optician and subsequently the pair of them entered their profession during the First World War. I wonder how they would feel to know that they were the geniture of a surprising number of medical descendants. The common theme in my ancestors was their shared commitment to the application of science and technology to human well-being.

Little now remains of the details of these brothers' personal history, which sadly is not surprising. Mine has not been a family that spoke much about its past, and as children we knew little of our origins. It was a Catholic and almost Victorian upbringing of 'being seen and not heard'. My father was a reticent and inaccessible character who was emotionally convincing in his belief system that a pessimist is a man in possession of all of the facts. He was rigidly right wing in his views and reluctant ever to explain his position or justify it, but only angrily to pontificate. I wanted to know more – to be enlightened about the genesis of these views – but he remained buttoned up, and the nearest I got to any explanation was when my mother let it slip in a sentence or two that he had had a tough and uncompromising upbringing in a severe and unemotional household. He never talked to us about anything: his only concept of a conversation was to give orders, or to enforce discipline. Maybe that was partly why he became an anaesthetist where he felt there was no need for him to converse much with anybody. All that was required was the briefest of verbal interventions before his patient was asleep, and unlike any son, completely under his control.

I did not find out until an adult that my paternal grandfather was born and raised in London, close to the docks, where his father was an artisan carver of jet. I can only conclude that their common interest in science came from a disciplined schooling. I am also aware that my father, the senior of the three sons, was placed under great pressure to achieve early academic success, leaving school at the age of 14, already with all his qualifications, though still too young to enter medical school, as the Second World War loomed. He had attended Finchley Grammar School, a Catholic educational establishment. Even though we lived nearby his old school, I was sent away to a Jesuit boarding school in Lancashire. Stonyhurst College provided me with a committed and rigorous religious upbringing. We attended Mass every morning, with evening prayers in the chapel as well as the service of Benediction on both Saturday and Sunday and our timetable, academic as well as sport, was constructed around those religious services. Every class began with the boys standing for prayer, every item of written work would be prefaced with the letters AMDG – *ad maiorem dei gloriam* – to the greater glory of God, and completed LDS – *laus deo semper* – praise to God always. On each of the weekday mornings there was a 20-minute period of 'morning studies' at which we would learn, and be tested on, sections of the catechism, which after three years at the prep school we could all recite by heart. Despite this deep involvement in the Catholic religion I did not receive or ever find the gift of faith. I could acknowledge the history of the church but my belief was confounded at the mystery of transubstantiation – the conversion of bread and wine in the mass into the body and blood of Christ – that then had to be consumed! I could follow that the mass might be an allegory of the Last Supper ('Do this in memory of me'), but I was uncertain about the cannibalism element, let alone the insistence that the bread was the body of Christ, which was, and is, patently nonsense.

Despite my cynicism, I never lost reverence for Catholicism and indeed it has followed me into my professional life where I have never failed to honour those who sacrificed their lives in taking Holy Orders. When I first entered general practice I looked after an order of nuns, taking charge of their medical care when about 30 of them lived in a convent in central London and eventually ushering each of them off the planet when their time came. I was also appointed to take care of the Jesuits at Farm Street church, their headquarters in Mayfair, as well as the secular priests living on the campus of Westminster Cathedral and even the Pope when he came to London in 1982. Despite my lack of religious conviction and involvement, I considered it a privilege to take care of these men and women, nearly all of whom, in my experience, have been noble and devoted individuals.

In childhood I only ever saw my father on weekends, and I can still remember one unique Sunday when he took me to his father's optician premises, where most unusually we rooted around inside of an outhouse where I even found a simple but effective microscope. I then spent the afternoon, with my father cleaning it, which now I remember as being one unusual moment of intimacy between father and son. The mechanism and lenses were intact, although much of the metal was corroded. Additionally, there was a wooden case containing glass microscope slides, many of them cracked or broken, but some of them were still intact. I also discovered samples of various insect and botanical specimens preserved under cover slips. At his instigation we found ourselves looking at living microorganisms from pond water, and it was I think, looking back through time, this early and shared experience that galvanized me into an interest in science and biology and my focus to what goes on *inside* of things. Perhaps, it is only now, as I record the nostalgia of that unusual day, once upon a time, that I am able to attribute to it the importance that I did not then know it would have upon my life.

When at school, many years later, we started to learn sciences, I had a sense of superiority and confidence as I found that I had already got a head start. Engagement with the study of science was the start of my pursuit towards medicine, ultimately it was all about my fascination with how things work, what goes on inside of things; and in particular inside of the human body. Dissection at school, first the dogfish, then the rabbit, later the frog, brought all this alive to me. All I wanted to do from then on was to obtain a place at medical school and be given permission to dissect a cadaver.

As a medical student I came under no influence from my father about what direction I should take. He only ever pushed me to get qualified quickly and not to hold back and waste time as he saw it by stopping off on the way to collect a BSc. degree, which was an option that was offered to those of us who were seen to be doing well, but which he saw only as an unnecessary and expensive delay. I graduated in 1973 when general practice – numerically GPs are the single greatest specialty in medicine – was only taught by apprenticeship. Doctors who had spent some years as junior hospital residents in a variety of posts would accept employment as assistants to Partners in established NHS practices and after a year in such a post would be considered fit for a partnership in their own right. The Vocational Training Act of 1980 changed all that.*

Primary care, or general practice, now emerged as a desirable career option along with the days of it being regarded as second

---

*   The idea was to accept postgraduates, who had completed their year as a house surgeon and house physician, on to a three-year rolling programme of four six-month junior-hospital-doctor posts in diverse specialties with two six-month posts as a GP trainee under the tutelage of a general practitioner who was designated as a trainer and additionally paid as such. At the end of three years the doctor would pass out as a fully trained general practitioner and during those three years there was an underpinning of a once weekly half-day seminar spent on specific GP training and an academic industry evolved to identify and teach the special skills peculiar to primary care, with senior lecturer and professorial posts in general practice now being created. This was all very worthy, and gave credence to the establishment of the Royal College of General Practitioners created by a private non-NHS GP in 1952.

best being over, and thus increasing the number of young doctors competing as never before for GP posts in their rush to avoid the chaos of repeated attempts at reorganization within the NHS. General practitioners at least had the freedom of being a set of independent subcontractors to the State and despite the fact that there was only a monopoly employer, the GP was able to retain that independence, free of most governmental micro-management. At that still-idealistic time there was relative freedom to do what seemed best for the patient.

Over the years some changes have been exerted; some entirely proper and sane, some less so. The NHS doctors in negotiations always with their eye on their incomes have sold themselves short, at least in terms of conducting medical care in an idealized patient-centred way. An insane change has been the introduction of a new contract for GPs in 2004 enabling their withdrawal from 24-hour, seven-day commitment. The GPs gasped at their own triumph in losing less than 10 per cent of their total emolument while dropping their true commitment down to office hours: no nights, no weekends. The doctors post-rationalize that forcing patients to consult them only at their surgeries in office hours makes for greater efficiency, greater accuracy, and better healthcare. Superficially, this looked to be a change for the good but for the patients it has been a disaster. The move away from house calls and 24-hour commitment is reflected in reduced commitment, skill and care by GPs in the home care of the chronically sick. Now I witness palliative care of the dying and the continuing care of elderly chronic sick discharged from hospital becoming the province of dedicated nursing teams that the government has been forced to evolve. These palliative-care responsibilities used to be a crucial part of any GP's daily life. The consequence of this amputation of responsibility for GPs is that they are becoming de-skilled. Today, young GPs, whether NHS or private, that I meet are unable to provide this critical care as they feel they no longer have what is now 'deemed' to be the relevant experience which was once a professional duty, or even a sacred *rite de passage*, conducted since time immemorial by family doctors.

The upshot of the post-2004 (contract) era is that NHS GPs have inadvertently commenced a process of marginalization, where they are no longer the team leaders but they have become another cog in a machine and are no longer the governors, the orchestrators, of care in the community. What has been lost in these few precious years is that most subtle ingredient of healthcare, continuity. There is a great premium on continuity as it is vital to the patients to know at a critical time in life that one professional individual knows their personal history, which goes far beyond the simple summation of a tonsillectomy, an appendectomy, a broken arm, hay fever, short sightedness, or terminal disease.

I argue that human beings have that need, especially when they are vulnerable and possibly regressed through their disease for the need for an omniscient guide, and that it should be the current and future role of the GP. Although he may not be there night and day, weekday and weekend as he used to be, he must remain as the backstop of wisdom: to interpret and explain, to help convey judgement. Information is not knowledge, and though patients will glean what they may need from the web world of information what they most often need is balance of judgement in the face of an often confusing battalion of alternatives. As so many of us have learned in medicine, knowing what not to do can be the critical act as well as are the catastrophic implications of wrong decisions. As Jane's favourite medical cynic, Proust reminds us: 'For each illness that doctors cure with medicine, they provoke 10 in healthy people by inoculating them with the virus that is a thousand times more powerful than any microbe: the idea that one is ill.'

DOCTORS DISSECTED

What are the attributes that might define a good doctor for modern man? No longer availability (he's not), affability (it is of no matter) or ability (taken for granted); but it must of course include trust and experience and so it is worth examining the facets of medical interventions that create trust. And here the wheel turns full circle. The trust that a mother has when her doctor handles her eight-week-old baby and gives the first injections is built when she is under his care as a younger woman, a teenager even; later, newly married she sees him when first pregnant and maybe at times during her pregnancy. Trust builds from the experience of a series of positive interventions combined with continuity of care. What every one of us needs is a keynote contact in medicine in whom we have a sense of trust which is the springboard for the affirmation of all knowledge about care: what referrals are right, what tests are safe or not, whether NICE-published* guidelines are reliable or biased towards cost-saving. Though my worry about the world of guidelines is that a move in that direction will initiate a re-shaping of the training of doctors in an unhealthy way so that political thought and action come to alter the course of medical scientific thought. Already, super-specialization has removed the general surgeon and general physician from the arena: the pressures of appraisal, revalidation, relicensing and corralling specialists are preventing us from involvement in anything but our precise and narrow sphere of activity. This is not always a good thing. In an environment where a patient sees a different specialist for hip, or knee, or elbow, who is in charge when it comes to major trauma, or systemic disease?

To answer my question, I have come to the conclusion that there is not a gene that determines vocation: it is not about brain or emotions, or anything innate. What a medical career is about is the melding of attitude, aptitude, and exposure to the thought patterns of what a life in medicine looks like, or is about. Despite popular belief, medical science is not hard, but there is a lot of

---

*   National Institute for Health and Care Excellence.

it. Considerable commitment, if not devotion, is always required involving application and determination regardless of whether one chooses a medical career out of a sense of vocation, or a desire for status and security. It is this that makes the study of medicine, if not its practice, an all-enveloping lifestyle choice. The breadth of knowledge, the continual evolution and development, the interplay between physiology, psychology and social factors, are all demanded throughout a medical training and a medical life. Nothing is the equivalent of the many years of experience that also have to be spent at the coalface before a young person can grasp what his intended medical life is really all about. My colleague George Lewith puts it so well.

> I learnt as a young houseman that in order to be a doctor you need to completely absorb yourself in medicine and only through hard work does medicine become part of you, it absolutely has to become part of your every fibre. I learnt to train myself to get up at 3 am, it becomes like riding a bike, a reflex – you know – in your bones, when you have seen so much that however tired you are, however knackered you are, you can just focus on the patient for a short time and know whether there's a serious problem which you can identify because it's a combination of having seen it so often and having it drilled into you when you were tired and having made mistakes, it just becomes part of you.

If there is no gene and it is mainly down to selection based on socio-environmental factors, what does that say about what and how our future doctors will evolve given the changing demographic, the changing environment, and the changes in social factors? Does it matter? Is there anything special about the role of the healer in 21st-century life, or has the idea of the doctor as a healer, rather than only as a scientist become an illusion, now that medicine is driven by an addiction to studies of molecular phenomena, and scientific objectivity?

DOCTORS DISSECTED

The idea of a gene for medicine is metaphorical, as is the concept of viruses in computers: it is an analogy. It is not a gene in the sense of an encoded script in the DNA of ourselves such as is found for red hair, or allergy, or haemochromatosis. It is not preordained in the child at birth, but it is part of nurture and environment nevertheless. The set of required attitudes that may have become ingrained through exposure in childhood so that the offspring of doctors often appear to be drawn innately to the study of medicine, much more so, than the tendency of the children of architects to be architects or engineers to be engineers or farmers to be farmers, or intriguingly dentists to be dentists. Yes, there is an additional extra ingredient somewhere there, which it would be difficult to deny is a contributory factor. Maybe it is because the vocational life aspects of the task of being a doctor cannot only be conveyed intellectually. The invisible responsibilities of being a doctor are often experienced within the domestic routines of the home: the impact upon the family on a daily basis is conveyed to the children of medical practitioners and somehow the developing personality – which is where DNA does come in – absorbs that.

I want to emphasize my opening thought: no one knows how to choose a medical student. The current philosophy seems to be that because the process is inevitably oversubscribed, the admissions officers must first of all go for academic perfection, and then attempt to distinguish between applicants at interview. The hope, or rather naive expectation must be that there will be a relationship, subsequently to be confirmed, between the identified qualities of young adults aged 18 or 19 years and the individuals who will emerge as general practitioners at the age of 30 or so, as half or more of all medical students will now become GPs.

Are medical practitioners a class apart? Are they different from professionals in other walks of life because of a difference of degree, or a difference of kind? If it is a difference of kind, is that due to an inherited trait, or is this is the result of a metamorphosis that has occurred during their long training? That metamorphosis could be a Damascene moment, a cognitive shift due to insights gained during the apprenticeship and that may be why the long medical apprenticeship is so important, for much of what is learned cannot be gained in any classroom, with or without role play by actors, which is the current trend. Even the word apprentice is now suppressed, and we can probably only venture to use the word mentor, whereas my own training has been defined by my mentors. Some of those moments of life changing emotional impact occurred during my six years of training: a *rite de passage* can be identified whose successful completion must inevitably change the students' attitudes, feelings, and their approach to medicine.

The first of these is dissection. At the age of 18 I walked into the dissecting room at University College, London with considerable trepidation. This is what I had striven to achieve since that afternoon in my childhood, and yet I felt completely unworthy of my position and as if everybody else present already had acquired some innate knowledge. I was terrified that I would be unequal to the task. I took up station with five others, sitting on high stools around the cadaver with which we developed an intimate relationship over the next 12 months. One of those is now an eminent and senior psychoanalyst; one is a senior lecturer in pharmacology at a teaching medical school, one was a GP until his mid fifties and has now abandoned medicine for a career as a professional photographer and artist. The last member of the group is lost to me.

The dissection room had 20 or 30 corpses on glass-topped trolleys, each covered in a white sheet, lying under brilliant fluorescent lighting. There was an overwhelming smell of formalin preservative and a sweeter smell of corpse. The corpse that was allocated to my group was female, skeletally thin and weighing maybe 45 kilos, elderly, ancient even, and with wisped, grey hair. A death-mask grimace returned our stares. None of this seemed either shocking or alarming to any of us, I sense that we took it in our stride as if to declare that we, as medical students, had no problem with the impact of our extraordinary setting.

The emotional heat we experienced was more about that every *viva* had to be passed, rather than the shock of our proximity to those corpses. I had never seen, apart from my mother in the bathroom 10 or more years earlier, a naked woman. Our coping mechanism became a raunchy bravado, dosed with considerable black humour, and a rapidly emerging easy familiarity with those female medical students in our group every one of whom seemed just as implacable and bullet proof as the boys. (Medical schools had had a compulsory intake of 50 per cent female students from two years prior to the time of my own admission.) Four days later we sat around the corpse undergoing our first viva voce examination: a question and answer session on the precise anatomy of the forearm and hand. Our grilling was conducted by a doctor who had taken time out from his clinical duties to study anatomy himself in greater detail, in preparation for becoming a surgeon.

Our daily dissection sessions were interleaved with anatomy lectures, physiology and biochemistry lectures, practical laboratory work, and a morning spent every week in the histology room examining slides of human tissues under microscopes. The academic weight of our first year was considerable, and had to be taken at a rapid pace. Every evening was spent studying and by the first major exams at 18 months, genetics, pharmacology and psychology had been added to anatomy, physiology and biochemistry. None of these subjects was very difficult intellectually but it was a huge volume of work.

After two years, we were examined in 20 or more papers, which terminated our grounding in basic sciences. Our group now moved on to what was then described as the clinical part of the course, and we were introduced to what were called 'teaching firms'. A group of four or five students would be attached to a consultant and his retinue of senior registrar, registrar and house officers. The day was spent sitting in Outpatients, listening to the consultant, or his registrars taking histories and examining patients, while simultaneously holding a discourse with the students. On surgical firms we experienced our next *rite de passage*, which included attendance in the operating theatre, and equally dramatically the moment of being present at a normal vaginal birth.

While on the medical firms we would attend patients on the wards, and witness the chaos surrounding the management of cardiac arrest and other trauma. Truly, it was an apprenticeship in every sense, the main task of the students, apart from being ever present and hoping to catch an opportunity to pick up exposure to some unpredictable event or another, was to take blood from the patients each morning after the houseman, the most junior of the hospital doctors, had written up the forms. The decision about what tests should be done were usually taken during the ward round on the previous day, when our entire retinue would drift from one bed to the next while the consultant, or the registrar would teach. After this, the drama of being on my first surgical 'firm', which comprises the consultant, his registrar and the junior doctors, meant that I had spent three months of which several hours of each day were in the operating theatre where I listened, observed and was transfixed by the unrehearsed human dramas of surgery.

A poignant and equally emotional and draining experience was the pathology 'firm', which also lasted for three months: some of it was in the form of a classroom activity when at least half a day each week was spent working at a microscope. Slowly, we learnt to identify the characteristics of diseased tissue at a cellular level, which is the process of histopathology. Another half day of each week was spent in the laboratory, again with a microscope, learning about blood cells, bone marrow, identifying leukaemias and other conditions, which become almost magically visible when inspecting blood films on glass slides.

My account makes it sound like a lot of work to absorb, but think how little teaching there really was when maybe we received 12 classes in practical haematology to fit us up for a life in medicine and another 12 classes in our introduction to histopathology. How would I cope if I found myself stranded in the depths of a third world country with little or no support, a diagnosis to make and a Victorian microscope sitting there mocking me? But then there was an implicit group assumption that this would never be our destination, although this year I have visited, not without difficulty, Bhutan. During my stay I was asked by a healthcare assistant, with only two years of training, in a village 65 miles from the nearest road where no visitor had been seen since 1980 to show him how to diagnose urinary infections using a microscope. In 1970 we all realized, as we gathered in those labs that none of us, well almost none, would ever work in isolated communities in the third world. We already knew that more than half of us would be GPs with fully-staffed services always available in the nearest District General Hospital. What we were learning was not so much the intimate detail necessary to the specialist, as the right approach, the critical training of those enquiring but sceptical attitudes that are so essential in diagnostic medicine and most importantly the notion that medicine is ever changing, ever advancing, where the important factors are to know where to look for information, and how to go about obtaining it.

While studying on the pathology firm there were two daily rituals. At 10 am, each day we would attend one or two, or sometimes three post-mortem examinations. This was a shocking and brutal process of immersion compared to the delicate and finessed way we had dissected a corpse in our first two years.

MARTIN ASKS...

Taking less than half an hour the pathologist would open a body, remove the brain, the lungs, the heart, all of the abdominal organs, the tongue, larynx in one bloody chunk with each part – or set of parts – being dunked, without ceremony, into large stainless steel bowls of preservative formalin. Around 20 students, mostly 20 years of age, sat watching this in a tiered semi circular lecture theatre, curved around the dissection table. The professor of morbid anatomy and pathology paced the floor, dressed in a full-length rubber apron and white rubber boots; as he lectured, he splashed us with drips of formalin. Deftly, he sliced a liver, which he held aloft in one hand, while balancing a 12-inch carving knife in the other, as he demonstrated to us the appearance of cirrhosis – 'The word means tawny' – I still hear him saying. In the same way, he sliced into the brain to reveal the site of a haemorrhagic stroke, or the heart to show the scarred myocardium from damage due to ischemic heart disease – with fatty deposits in the arteries immediately apparent – as he cut the sections through the muscle of the heart that was once someone's life. This was the crudest yet most informative of processes that I was to be inducted in. It was primitive in a medieval sort of way, and all was conducted in a haze of formalin and with an aroma of faeces.

At 1.30 pm each day, during the second half of the lunch hour, 40 or 50 people would cram in to the morbid anatomy theatre for each of the morning's post-mortems to be presented by the houseman responsible for the care of the patient when they were admitted. His role was to describe the history taking, what diagnosis was then reached, and what had happened to lead to the death of that individual. This ritual was followed by the description, or perhaps it was more like a sentence, of the findings at post-mortem by the pathologist. My heart was usually in my mouth as I was forced to watch the discomfort of someone else being publicly put on the spot, being shown up for being incompetent, although the whole process was utterly gentlemanly and non confrontational. So often the houseman's diagnosis had been completely wrong, or at the best, only partial, or there had been additional undisclosed pathology. There was never any remonstration, only a solemn and serious reckoning of events: everything was about learning and not about any apportionment of blame or criticism. Consultants, senior registrars, housemen and students would be present if the post-mortem involved a patient of that firm. There would be brief discussion between all parties and sometimes some clear, firm, and even harsh words were to be heard being exchanged between the senior registrar and his more junior colleagues. I learned more from that process than I ever learned in lectures, tutorials, or maybe even in the operating theatre.

One day, when there had been no deaths in the preceding 24 hours in Westminster Hospital, our morning session still did not lack for teaching material. The pathologist arrived, late and breathless, explaining that he had come from Vincent Square, the site of Westminster Children's Hospital, which was a 10-minute walk. He swung his brown leather briefcase up on to the porcelain post-mortem slab, with its drainage grooves and plughole for body fluids and formalin, and opened it. He removed his sandwiches (wrapped in greaseproof paper as it was before the days of cling-film), a book or two, some piles of exam papers he was marking, and finally the body of a tiny baby, completely naked, not even wrapped in a towel or sheet. He proceeded to dissect it, surrounded by the contents of his briefcase, without even donning a gown or any gloves. The baby looked like a porcelain doll, not emaciated, not ill, or ravaged by IV lines or surgical incisions. We discovered that it had died just after birth of a cerebral haemorrhage. I think that even those of us who were especially case hardened from two or three years at medical school, the rituals of dissection, the brush with death

MARTIN ASKS...

(I liked to think I was, being a deeply hardened cynic after eight years at a tough Jesuit boarding school) were affected deeply by the experience of that morning.

I can only think of one other moment as a student or junior doctor, which has had quite the same and lasting impact. I was now working in Casualty and was sent to escort a relative to the mortuary to identify a young man who had been killed in a motorcycle accident near the hospital. The fridges were arranged like a row of filing cabinets, with each drawer containing one corpse. I pulled open the correct one – there he was – not in a shroud, but fully dressed, in shirt and tie, and still wearing a green waxed cotton jacket. The corpse was about my age and on his wrist a watch was still ticking as he lay dead in that drawer. Even now I think about him, even though I never knew any details of his life, only his name, his age, and how he died. I especially think of him when I am far from home on a big bike, I like to think that he keeps me alive.

We followed on from pathology to a part of our course that was even more dramatic, as the most exciting moment of all was my first attendance in the operating theatre, which I still recall as a moment of intense drama and considerable fascination in which every one of my senses was assaulted and enlightened. The cliché is that the medical student is expected to faint but I was far too excited, and from the first minute I was utterly engaged by the drama of the spectacle. Equally, I was rather nervous as emotions run high, tempers are short, and it was all too easy to be standing in the wrong place, or brush clumsily against something that was sterile and should not be touched.

The double doors from the anaesthetic room burst open and the trolley with the patient rushed through and was parked parallel to the operating table. A porter at one end and the anaesthetist at the other then lifted the patient off the trolley, while a pole on either side is withdrawn from the canvas runner upon which the patient is lying. These poles, unceremoniously, then being dumped on the trolley, which is whisked away. All of this time the patient has not been breathing as they were anaesthetized in another room, where a nasal catheter or tube was inserted into the windpipe, and now at that moment of transfer to the operating table, a necessary disconnection from the ventilator takes place. The anaesthetist quickly adjusts the connection between the anaesthetic machine supplying oxygen and the anaesthetic gas, until once again I saw that the chest of the patient was rising and falling. Instantly, the theatre porter strips off the gown from the patient who now lies naked on the operating table. Brilliant lights are illuminated, while the registrar, or the theatre sister paints the abdomen with bright iodine. The patient is then clad in green fabric sheets, leaving only a tiny area exposed for the surgeon to open up the abdomen. The surgeon advances from the corner of the room where he has been washing his hands and, now in sterile gloves, he joins his registrar. There is a further bustle of activities as the theatre sister nestles her trolley of instruments at either side of the patient's legs and feet, the anaesthetist is now engrossed at the head of the table, and everybody now huddles shoulder-to-shoulder, eyes focused on to the abdomen as the surgeon mutters to the anaesthetist, 'Okay to start?' Even before the reply is granted, a scalpel cuts more then an inch deep, an incision which provokes yellow fat to burst out of the wound and blood to pour. Swabs are called for, and interestingly the bleeding seems to be less than I imagined. Diathermy (which is electrically induced heat) is applied, and accompanied with the fizzing, bubbling sound, is the smell of cooking and burning. This, I thought, is what I came to see.

A virgin spectator, I was assaulted by this panoply of sensations: what is routine, a daily and constant task for the consultant, his registrar, the anaesthetist, and the theatre sister, was an emotionally overwhelming experience for me. Not quite green, after over a year dissecting a cadaver, I was still unprepared. I had anticipated none of the smells or noises and was naively expecting silence, tension and reverence. The surgeon and his assistant were, I recall, chatting about last night's TV, the rugby on Saturday, or illicit activities between members of staff; all intercut with terse orders for a McIndoe, diathermy, sucker, or clip, another clip, tie, 'cut there', or wet pack...

Those first operations I attended as a student were the lists of a general surgical team which meant abdominal surgery: resections of the rectum, or colon, or stomach, gall bladder removal, prostatectomy, aortic aneurysm repairs, thyroid surgery. This was all dramatic surgery, the more delicate procedures were reserved for the later firms to which we were attached as final year students: ENT, eye surgery, gynaecology but by then we were hardened off, and some of our group already thoroughly uninterested in surgery and heading for cardiology, psychiatry or chest medicine. I was excited even inspired by the long hours standing at operating tables watching routines, which by now were familiar.

Apart from dissection, witnessing surgery remains the singular thing that has most separated me from everyone who has not had this experience. It is difficult to find an analogy, it is not like getting married although that also changes your world-view, but marriage, or partnership is more of an emotional and psychological learning curve. There are so many sensory aspects to theatre that it is not possible to fantasize about in advance and seeing surgery on the television can never replicate physical inhalations of the aural and olfactory sensations that surge around that exclusive enclosure. As I have described we started with major abdominal surgery, it was not tonsils, or ears which are comparatively refined stuff, it was very visceral and thus in a way, it felt secret. What are your viscera? Who thinks about their own viscera? They include your liver, spleen and yards of gut and it is all very noisy indeed. To begin with, it feels as if nobody else outside of theatre has got any idea about what this secret club is that you are allowed into. Society used to be more familiar with visceral displays of the criminal corpses that were quartered and hung as the consequences of public executions until the 19th century. There are still earthy people in the 'country set' who are used to seeing a sheep or large deer eviscerated but even that does not make provision for another dramatic almost magical component in surgery, which is that the anaesthetized and inanimate body in front of you has to be repaired and then put back together again. I was fascinated, always have been and shall be, by that idea. I have always been drawn towards trying to ascertain what is going on beneath any surface and one can be more precise with surgery. Yes, it is this fascination with what phenomenon is being exposed beneath the skin surface – and the patients, quite literally, are exposed when they enter theatre to be opened up – which made me consider becoming a surgeon.

On that first day I did not know that the patient was going to be brought in, stark naked, on the trolley. It is at first quite shocking, this absence of discretion as everything is ripped off, although nothing is prurient and nobody is interested in nudity. As patients we imagine that we are covered up by all those green towels and things but really the operating gown that is ceremoniously put on is just to reassure the patient as it is removed again as soon as they are unconscious; being no more than an aesthetic nicety. Someone peels back the blanket and the patient is lying naked except for their white surgical stockings and those iodine daubings. The surgeon comes forward and cuts through the abdominal wall. It has become less dramatic now because as with keyhole surgery everyone in theatre is watching a screen. To begin with I used to wonder if a patient would wake up again and there were other thoughts like whether they would be in excessive pain, which they are not because any wound that is made when you are anaesthetized will not hurt as much as a wound which is inflicted when conscious. It is the same with animals who recover much faster because of the absence of any advance cognitive anxiety. Yes, there is a lot of speculation to begin with and then it becomes routine and you stop thinking in such personalized ways. The humanizing impact drops off surprisingly quickly.

As students we had a sense of trepidation, standing well out of the way with a reverence I previously reserved for serving as altar boy in church services. The anaesthetist is completely in charge for a few minutes as monitoring systems are connected, intravenous lines checked and running, and everything put in place for the surgeon and assistant to approach the table gloved and gowned, the scalpel already cutting deep through the skin and yellow fat bulging. 'If you must,' quipped the anaesthetist, setting the tone for an hour or two of jokes, puns, ribald stories, scandal about other staff members, periodically interrupted for a moment of concentration when the going got tricky but mostly it was a time of levity if not frank hilarity. Later on my wife always said that this apparently facile schoolboy activity – black humour and all – was reasoned by the awesome responsibility of the job and there may be something in that.

For years we have seen published articles about the health benefits of humour decreasing the perception of pain, and laughter even protecting against high blood pressure and how a sense of humour keeps us healthy and makes us live longer, helping to create feelings of well-being, lowering blood pressure by reducing spasm in blood vessels. We hear from a medical researcher that gallows humour about death and serious medical drama, laughter and jokes among the medical professionals, may not be as inappropriate, unethical or unprofessional as it might seem. Treating serious or painful material in a light hearted way serves as a support mechanism, aiding coping, increasing team bonding, and easing tension. My colleague at work in the practice told me as I write this that when he worked on the AIDS unit locally, in the early days as that epidemic emerged, the staff would pirouette around in the office singing 'another one bites the dust' when one of the patients died. Shocking, but there is an invisible line beyond which humour cannot pass: joking about a patient in front of them or the family is unethical and must never happen.

Later, when I became a house surgeon, I was unusually fortunate that I did quite a lot of surgery on my own because Professor Ellis, the consultant I worked under happened to have a female registrar that he did not get on with. He was known to be misogynistic and this registrar, who was Catholic, refused to do the vasectomies. She very much got on the wrong side of him, in fact it was commonly known that he really, really did not like her and so he would allow me to perform the vasectomies and the hernias and then in Outpatients he expected me to do all sorts of things also completely unaided, like the cysts. Because I had watched major surgery Ellis just expected me to go in and get on with it with only a nurse helping. There were anxious moments when there was just too much blood happening in the wrong place, or when I was presented with an extra large cyst, which I had struggled to get out and which I didn't then know if I would be able to suture the skin flaps back together. In surgery you can quickly feel out of your depth. I knew that even if I did not manage to pursue surgery as a career I would have six fascinating months ahead as a house surgeon after I qualified and I would never be the same again. To become a part of this living theatre, it changes you.

Forever.

2
JANE WANTS
TO KNOW

March 2010

My last patient of the day, by coincidence a young Iranian obstetrician who had suffered with postnatal depression and who had come back to see me to celebrate her long journey to Membership of the Royal College of Obstetricians has just left. As we say 'Goodbye' and I wait for Martin's arrival, I follow her steps into the night. Moonlight falls across the Georgian rooftops of Gloucester Place, which was built in 1810 and on to the marble threshold where I consult as a psychotherapist.

I enjoy the chill imagining of some of my ghostly neighbours. No. 99 was Elizabeth Barrett's first London home; John Godley, the founder of Canterbury, New Zealand, lived at No. 48; and opium-smoking Wilkie Collins lived at No. 65, where he wrote *The Moonstone* and where the same moon still shines above the street. Edward Lear and Anthony Trollope lived but a stone's throw around the corner. Across the evening at No. 50 visitors are arriving at the double frontage and portico grandeur of the Theosophy Society, some of whom are hoping to find their grail, whatever that may be, and others to find the spirits of their loved or departed. I imagine Madame Blavatsky a swathed and chiffon-pastel shroud, pause on the balcony to summons in the sceptical and faint-hearted; now the romance and trot of Elizabeth Barrett's Penny Post carriages delivering love letters to Browning come unbidden to my ear.

DOCTORS DISSECTED

Martin arrives, always a few energetic minutes early. I like to think of him as an expectant crow (I have a childish tendency to attribute bird forms to human types, and some would argue that the crow has inordinate intelligence) tapping at my window. Dressed slender in a three-piece, he sips his usual brew of two parts English Breakfast and one Lapsang Souchong.

While we are waiting for tea to brew I notice his cuff links – these wrists are never buttoned – composed of chrome and ceramic, before my gaze is drawn towards his limber and competent hands, which evoke those of a pianist or a surgeon, and do not seem to belong to a 60-year-old. I intend to begin by finding out more about what it *felt* like for Martin to become a patient when he donated a kidney to his ex-wife, Glynis. Hitherto, he has not provided a word about his feelings when he discovered his kidney donation was sabotaged by an unacknowledged surgical incompetence. After all kidneys do not come in bunches and now that his stepson Ben also needs a transplant it must feel horribly wasteful. It is not easy to persuade Martin to focus on feelings.

Well, I was determined not to behave like a patient and to take it all in my stride, but donating a kidney involves a lot of medicalization. I had only had one previous and brief admission for knee surgery when my wife Glynis had not even noticed I had been in hospital for the night. Well, she probably had, but her own domestic landscape was one of such constant hospital visits and having her creatinine levels measured was like you or I going to the hygienist. One morning you have to have a kidney X-ray and the next it's an arteriogram when they stick a walloping needle into your groin, you have to go in overnight and they shave off all your pubic hair, and it's all quite frightening even for a 42-year-old doctor. I was determined not to be one of those extra neurotic doctor patients, so I just looked interested and talked the doctors through the procedures.

JANE WANTS TO KNOW

We were admitted to the Middlesex Hospital together and parked in our single-sex wards but then we got dressed again and eloped out to Harrods and had lunch in a restaurant full of ladies in hats. It was incredibly poignant because there was a serious chance Glynis might die and a teeny-weeny one that I might and then we went back to hospital in a taxi and returned to our respective wards and took our clothes off again. Yes, we did a bit of visiting of each other in our dressing gowns. The next day they took me down to theatre first because they had to take my kidney out and then they brought Glynis down and had to bung my kidney into her. Yes, it is a much bigger operation for the donor because they had to remove my kidney off my aorta, which means making a very deep hole whereas for the recipient, although they are already the critically ill patient, it is a simpler operation, where you just have to pop the kidney into their groin.

I remember waking up with a catheter in my bladder, which I dreaded, a line in my neck and a drip thing in my arm. They had moved me next to the nurses' station and I was just lying there connected up to tubes and things, Glynis was in another ward and we didn't have any contact with each other for a few days, not until somebody wheeled her in to see me. Anyway, I was lying there next to the nurse station when the sister said, 'We have a call from University College Hospital for you,' and she stretched out the phone to me. I don't think I had really sat up until then. It was a registrar who had rung my office and been told that I was at the Middlesex, and he had assumed that I was visiting a patient, 'We've got a Father Anthony Meredith here. We are told he is your patient and we need an urgent letter.' I told him I was a patient on the ward but he still said they would send a medical student and asked me to dictate the letter to him for an urgent neurology referral. The sister didn't intervene so I was showing off and I did it. It was all a bit shaky and I said to the student,

'I'm probably much worse than your patient.' I went home on the fifth day and because I had been fit before surgery I recovered quickly but I wasn't supposed to drive for a month so I walked over from Ladbroke Grove to see Glynis at the Middlesex every day for two months. She was still so ill but we knew the transplant hadn't taken after a couple of days when she lost it because of medical incompetency. She had been erroneously connected up and her renal vein had thrombosed, but nobody admitted to the incompetence, that was the worst thing for her of all, being lied to. It took years to find out the truth.

Did your father take any interest in such a serious procedure?

No, as I've said he didn't take interest in things outside of his own work. I think he would have thought I was mad to do such a thing, but he never spoke to me about anything. I think he thought it was a very dangerous thing to do but he did visit me once and he brought in a bottle for a single glass of champagne, in fact he brought two bottles and said, 'This is medicine.' That was as sweet as I can ever remember him being – it didn't come easy on him to visit, and my mother came with him.

Glynis was very ill after the transplant failed. She was only just managing before the surgery, vomiting several times a day and afterwards she had to stay in hospital because she had lost the kidney and when she came home we decided to start home dialysis. Dialysis is exhausting; there are two versions, haemodialysis in which you plug in and your blood goes through an electric machine but then there is also this sophisticated but simpler process called chronic ambulant peritoneal dialysis where you insert a rubber tube under your abdominal wall, yes it is just floating about your guts and the tube sticks out here and there is Elastoplast to keep it in place. There is also a big bag of fluid of two or three litres of stuff, it is a salty and sugary water brew and your peritoneal membrane allows all the toxins in the blood to diffuse across. After an hour or two you just run it out, like the bath and it comes out looking like urine. Yup, we did the dialysis two or three times every day. First of all you warm the fluids bag to body temperature in a microwave, else you get a shock putting all that cold stuff in but it meant that everywhere we went with two kids we had to take boxes of this fluid with us. By then Glynis was very good at it and sometimes she would do it in the car when we were going up to the country. She coped for 12 years until another kidney came along but it caused problems because you have still got this tube inside and it gets infected. It is pretty horrible and she got hernias and then at the very end we had no choice but to do conventional dialysis. We had moved both of our offices to a house in Ladbroke Grove so I could be in the house all the time and Glynis had her film company on the ground floor while I converted the basement into my consulting room and it all worked very well until I left the marriage.

You didn't have a family GP? Would you do that again with hindsight, would you so closely intertwine the professional and the emotional?

No, we didn't. I just gave the children that banana-flavoured antibiotic medicine, you remember don't you, when they had childhood infections. Probably not, no definitely not now, I tend to keep things separate, although my next partner – with whom I had two children – was a doctor. One day she said, 'Could you do a smear test for me?' She just hopped up on to the kitchen table and afterwards she said, 'That's much nicer than usual. That didn't hurt.' 'Of course it wouldn't hurt, it never hurts when I do it for anybody, I'm careful.' I remember that so clearly in my mind but then I don't think any other woman I was involved with would ever consider me doing a smear test but we were in practice together and we were so earthy going about our lives and it was just a practical thing, not a sexual thing. No, now I don't have anything at all to do with the management of the medical issues of the women in my life, or my other son Mylo, who is Cosmo's half-brother by a subsequent partner. I just tell them they look beautiful and refer them to a specialist but it is different when you are married and you have young children. Life is hard and you cut corners rather than queue up at the doctor's for your appointment. Today, it is not even regarded as good practice by the GMC if the partners in a practice look after each other.

Did this domestic background of critical illness in Glynis and potentially in your stepson Ben and then Cosmo make a difference when you had to deal with the 'heart sink' patients, otherwise known as timewasters, in your practice?

Yes, but I concealed any contempt that I felt for the hypochondriacs, the heart sink patients, but I often think like that in general, and anyway it is all an act. You put on your professional mask and you play a part. It is an important part, it's definitely a large part of me but it is still all an act. Don't you think that most of life is an act? I remember around that time a patient came in an immaculate suede jacket and dark glasses, just back from the Indian Ocean and he said, 'I'd like another week's holiday now, you know looking after the kids, it's not a real holiday.' I thought, 'Really, you don't know anything about anything when it comes to the stress and pressure of life' but I was very nice to him, and patient. He is still my patient now, 18 years on. You cannot take your mask off, no, but every now and again mine has slipped, and yes perhaps I do in some intimate relations. Here I am at weekends wearing a three-piece suit. Even in the country I wear a corduroy suit and waistcoat, whereas in the old days I wore jeans but I think they are a bit unbecoming in men of 60 and anyway the really old neighbours in Norfolk expect me to look the part when I visit and look after them at weekends. So I have grown into being a bit of an old fogey but it took a long while, I am quite a late developer.

You have explained that there were a lot of fatal illnesses in your family of origin and that your father's younger brother died after he followed in your father's footsteps to train at the Westminster Hospital.

My father never talked to me about his brother. He never talked to me about anything, ever. I call him aspergoid; there is no warmth in him, not a word ever. There is a strange thing, which I can't explain and I don't know if I will ever get to the bottom of it but in the spare bedroom in our house, my parents still live there, but in the spare bedroom is a bedside table. When I was 11 my sister and I were fiddling about and we found some letters tied up in ribbon. We thought we would look at them and they were from John, my father's dead younger brother, to my mother and we got into a bit of trouble about this. I don't know why he was writing but they must have been love letters all done up in ribbon. Was there some agenda between them? Could they have known each other, been lovers and he then died? But he was much younger than my father, there was 10 years between them, so we still don't know what it was about. John died from a teratoma of the testicle, which had metastasized to his lungs. My father was always examining our bollocks when we were children and yes he was always coming into the bathroom and examining our bollocks just checking us out but he was anxious.

Dad's other brother Henry developed a neurosis after John died and he had to see a psychiatrist because he was afraid of this cancer. He was an optician like my grandfather in Barnet, and quite unlike my father who was always such a professional star. He was just an optician; very Catholic, very religious and he had to be sedated for anxiety. When he was 65 he retired from work and in no time at all he got cancer of the testicle and died of it. Yes, he made it happen. Amazing, amazing. Father wouldn't go to Henry's funeral but he asked me, 'Do you want to go to Henry's funeral?' It was impossible for me to go, I was working in the NHS at the time. 'Well, I'm not going if you don't come, I'll only go with you.' He didn't go. My father said he thought all funerals were a waste of time and that he would prefer it if a laundry type shute opened in the wall. He doesn't like any expressions of emotion but now that he is demented and close to death he has been talking a lot about wanting to be buried and not to be burned and wanting to see a priest. Henry died and he had a son called Anthony, my first cousin who also died of cancer at 19. Anthony developed a painful shoulder – he had been working in a dartboard factory and they said he'd been playing too much darts and not working hard enough – but it was a liposarcoma of bone and he died of it when it metastasized to his lungs. He vomited, coughed up his blood and died on it. Such family tragedies but my father never spoke about them. I must go and talk to Mother about it, she is 80-plus but still very with it. She is much more amenable to talking even though we don't get on at all well, we never have, but I must speak to her before she goes batty too.

JANE WANTS TO KNOW

Although you rejected Catholicism early you do seem to have spent an unusual amount of time attending to prominent Catholics. Has their faith helped you to cope with the experiences of death that are your daily bread?

I always think that it is those people who have devoted themselves to their religious faith who are the worst when it comes to dying. I've looked after very many priests and no, no I've not learnt anything about readiness for death from them. They are the most anxious, the most hysterical and the hardest to control. I have often found it less distressing working with patients in the hospice. I imagine they are afraid they are going to find they have backed the wrong horse after all these years, although they won't know once they are dead, but there is very much that sense – when they are facing terminal illnesses – of it all being too late. Only Cardinal Hume died with grace, or peace. No, their faith didn't help many of them to die, not at all and it has often shocked me the way so many of them are all over the shop and much less composed than the hospice patients I looked after in St John and Elizabeth's Hospice. It shocked me and that is partly why I had to give them so much support, because if you are a priest who is dying prematurely of cancer and underneath it you are simply ridden with guilt about your inevitable sins and how many times you have masturbated, then it is very hard work to die. I was thinking about celibacy this morning. Oh, very taxing for me even to think about it. My first patient this morning was a Jesuit and I was thinking how hard must it be to live this celibate life, well half of them aren't, they have their own entertainments but some definitely are and it must be bloody difficult.

Then there are the nuns who can be very spiteful, competitive and hysterical. When I started looking after the 35 nuns of the Order of Mercy at St John's, they were all on Valium because the GP before me had kept them all on psychotropic drugs to keep them under control. The majority of them were neurotic and anxious, even hysterical and his solution was medication. Mine was to listen to them and so I learnt a lot about their feelings, and I particularly remember one of them. She was about 45 and had been there since she was 15 when she was sent over from Madeira. She had no choice; she was just the eighth daughter and it was her destiny to be sent off to a convent. Only the demented ones died well. They all got very dotty. I had never seen a dementia like my father's before because most people return to a second childhood but my father is angry, aggressive and anxious and he still wants to know whether I've managed to get a job. The nuns were just dozy and I didn't use any drugs. It was all very grand and Victorian, their accommodation I mean, and lovely too, but no wisdom to be found for me there. But you know, I also cannot believe what privilege I have had.

I am wondering, seeing that your father has been unsatisfactory as a father, who were your mentors, or the seminal influences in your life?

James Scobie, the retired GP who was the senior partner in the first NHS surgery where I was a GP trainee in 1974. He was very down to earth and practical, but he had to retire early because of health problems. When I got older and was in private practice, it was Sir Richard Bayliss at the Westminster Hospital, a physician who was always in my background. He was Physician to the Queen and I had been his houseman at Westminster Hospital where he also looked after all the neurotic wives of the other consultants but he was still a generalist in an area where people were becoming more specialized. He was also an endocrinologist. He elected me as a Fellow to the Royal College of Physicians after I had passed the Membership and then we would go to the Reform Club for lunch and I would present him with a problem case and he always backed me. He would come and give an opinion about a tricky patient in hospital. It was always very good to have that degree of backing from someone in indisputable authority. He died on the day of the Queen's Jubilee and the Queen sat down at her desk on that day and wrote a letter personally, although it was her 25th anniversary but she still wrote personally to Lady Bayliss. Yes, they were very different types of men: Scobie was a thinker, an adventurer but not an academic like Bayliss.

You love to use Latin words when you are talking about a diagnosis. It is like you might be speaking about a beautiful flower, and it seems to be habitual, but I don't hear many, or rather any other doctors I know doing that. When we were talking about genes you seemed to pluck 'haemochromotosis' out of the air like a butterfly. Why?

I don't know why I said that, Greek of course, not Latin but I don't know why I chose it. Haemo, of the blood, chromo is colouring, because you go rusty, what is happening here is a disorder of the blood, and it is quite an unusual thing but it just fell out of my mind. I suppose that is Bayliss' influence, it's something that he did it and I like it. I could have said the gene for haemophilia.

It is rather like people using Latin names for plants.

Yes, but that can be annoying too when someone says 'betula pendula' and I think why can't you just call it a silver birch. Gardeners do it to death. My mother only ever uses the Latin name for her plants, which I think makes her feel more important. I also feel so irritated about the dumbing down of medicine, the fact that people cannot name things. I don't think I say these things out of arseholeness but we should try and lift things up, not down. Sir Richard Bayliss and Prof Harold Ellis, perhaps the most famous surgeon of the 20th century, and now in his eighties, were both like that too. Prof Ellis is an East End Jew whose parents made wedding dresses and they lived near the London Hospital in Whitechapel Road and Ellis was proud of it. He started off as a very down to earth registrar in Sheffield. He used to say, 'Why do you do up the buttons of your white coat, Jones?' 'I don't know, sir.' 'It stops you getting shit on your tie.' That is just one Ellis aphorism. When he examined a patient who had had an operation for cancer he would tell us that the way you remember what to do in the follow up examination is to use the mnemonic LUMPS (liver, umbilicus, moving dullness, per rectum, supraclavicular nodes). There were loads of them and that was how he taught. He always used technical terminologies, we had to understand them, he wouldn't bring it down to a nursery school level and I still think it's important. The new generation are not interested in working or speculating in great detail whereas I'm only interested in the broadest paint strokes of diagnosis rather than the contemporary simplicity of general practice where GPs immediately make referrals when it is something that is not routine.

As I imagined, you were always competent with your hands, which brings us back to the excitement of your first day in theatre and why you are not a surgeon. I have the intuition that if your father had shown even a shred of interest in your development and success you might have been.

JANE WANTS TO KNOW

Yes, that is what I had come to medical school for. I probably should have been one but I couldn't bring myself to be doing more exams. Then guess what I did, I immediately did more exams. The MRCP examination is probably harder, but nobody gave me the endorsement that I needed to have the self-confidence to do surgery. I didn't have any support at all, although I was the only one in our year to get Honours in surgery and that is why Harold Ellis took me on as his houseman. All the other Ellis 'boys' are famous consultants now. Yes, perhaps being a surgeon would have suited me better because it is a skill, a craft and you don't have to wear a mask all the time, except in theatre. It is not an intellectual thing, and you are expected to be ruthless, you have to be, to be a good surgeon. I always say that surgeons are like Exocet missiles, but they do not always have good clinical judgement and you should only fire them when you have already found your target. It is no use doing heroic surgery if you don't also know when not to, and sometimes I have to protect my patients from them.

Father just said, 'Get a living and anyway you'll earn more as a GP.' He was wrong but he was angry with the way state medicine had turned out. If he had said, 'You should do surgery because you are very good with your hands, I have no doubt that you will do it well and you could also be an anatomy lecturer.' But he didn't, if he had I would have done it because I was very obedient then. My cousin John Scurr has done very well as a surgeon and his dad was an optician who was a more generous man, and perhaps a better father. I didn't have the self-confidence then and I was desperate to own a house and a car, I was quite materialistic, I still am really. So getting on was all about becoming a GP. I rather wish I had done surgery but so what, the grass is always greener. It gives me huge pleasure when I meet consultant surgeons of all sorts and colours and they need me to advise them and say, 'Is it safe for my wife to be on the pill, which one would you recommend?' I get great pleasure when I realize they do not have my breadth of knowledge that they are just focused on one thing and are entertained by the fact that I do know a bit about everything.

Can you recall first seeing a baby born?

Yes, I knew what was going to happen and where it was coming from but, firstly, I couldn't believe how shitty it was and, secondly, you cannot believe that the baby can get out but of course they do, because it's all so stretchy. I even remember from the hospital notes the house the woman lived in, and I can remember the midwife's face – she was freckly and looked like Aretha Franklin – and I can still remember her voice. She delivered the first birth and then I had to deliver the next one. We had to deliver 12 in a month. It is all bloody dramatic stuff and I can remember thinking this is quite difficult and it was like losing my virginity in a way, and in fact they both happened to me at the same time. I was a virgin when I went to medical school and then my father made me live at home during my training to save money until I had to go and live in Roehampton as all the students who were doing obstetrics had to live in. Immediately, I got laid by a fabulous Mauritian nurse! Yes, these beginnings definitely went together and it was also the moment that Jimi Hendrix died. I went on to work at St Mary Abbots Hospital, where Jimi had died. I remember a lot about that time, as there were all these emotionally shaking events like me shagging this Mauritian bird, rather ineffectually, well, effectually but ineffectually. I was 20 and about to be 21, it was May 1970, or April 1970. She was a beauty called Biddy Teelanah but then she moved on to somebody else, well she was something of a goer. After Nurse Biddy I knew what to do, well

I didn't not know what not to do, but I got more confident at both activities.

Sitting here now, drinking tea, what moment from all these beginnings comes back into a random focus?

Loads. Well, the first time I ever went to take blood at Westminster and the housemen said, 'This is a syringe, use a green needle and stick it in a vein and you put a tourniquet on and take blood, so off you go with your trays.' This is not a story about me, it is about Ken Rhodes, who was my quite good friend. We were told that first of all you pull the curtains round and you say, 'Hello Mrs. Smith I want to take your blood today,' except in those days we routinely took blood from every patient in the hospital every day. I heard Ken saying, 'Wake up Mr Riseborough, I've come to take your blood, Mr Riseborough.' I heard lots of slapping sounds on the shoulder and then I thought Ken's patient is dead. Mr Riseborough had died. The curtains were already drawn around his cubicle but nobody had told Ken and I just heard all this slapping happening behind closed curtains.

How harsh we were as students, we just laughed at everything, we coped with all the death by humour, there was nothing dignified or respectful. We had no teaching in ethics, or how to behave at all. We were told that we had to have a tie and white shirt with formal wear and to be clean but nobody talked to us about dignity. Or maybe they did and we blacked it out. Maybe the gallows humour is necessary to survive as it is a way of dealing with such darkness. As students either you go to bed with each other, or you get humorous, or you do both. You see people dying again and again. When I have to do a death certificate now I go through the stubs of my book, oh God it is so moving, you go through the stubs and you remember and you remember.

DOCTORS DISSECTED

After Martin left I needed pause to recover breath before I could go home. His thoughts still flamed across my room. My own had involuntarily returned to the subject of masks and specifically to what sort of mask he had been wearing throughout our conversation. Although, as he relaxed, he appeared relatively unmasked. The self is like a Russian doll: as you unbolt one segment there is always another, albeit smaller, or perhaps it is a larger segment of Martin's masked self that is left to undress…

I thought too, in contrast to the speed with which he moves, both mentally and physically, of his patience and how he enjoys explaining the inner mechanisms of how just about anything and everything works, including my recorder, or an undiscovered mechanism on my Apple, all of which terrify me. At times I sensed his ears expanding as he listened. Martin has small features but what he would call 'sticky out' ears about which he is self-conscious. Now, I am thinking that those ears, like a bat's, are listening, always listening out for rhythms of abnormal energy and how a doctor has to learn to develop both his eyes and ears and like a sniffer dog, his nose to suss out disease at a primal and intuitive level. When Martin says that he has 'seen it all' one knows that it is not an exaggeration. He has seen it all, and he also knows all there is to know about the uncertainties of medicine and life. In Martin's philosophy of life nothing can be assumed until it has been understood.

3
FIRST MEETING
WITH COSMO

March 2010

I suspected it would not be as easy to pin down Cosmo, who seems even busier than his father, to a meeting. However, he replied enthusiastically to my initial email saying enigmatically that he approved our book project as he thought: 'It would encourage my father to focus his ideas.' This initial enthusiasm seemed to coincide with a period of voluntary work with the Ambulance Service, in addition to his full-time employment on 'nights' in the hospital as a Junior Doctor along with his urgent job applications. Several subsequent emails remained unanswered until Martin tempted Cosmo to find the time to meet me with an offer to provide him en route to my office with a prescription for his chronic blood pressure medication which would save him a 'time wasting' visit to his GP. It was immediately clear that like his father, Cosmo was not keen on any time-wasting activities, including, somewhat disturbingly, taking care of his health.

My first thoughts, as I opened the door to Cosmo and his bicycle, despite it being a freezing March night was that he didn't have any outerwear over his light jumper, and how often this is the case with schoolboys and young men. His only concession to anything elemental was a battered safety helmet. I was taken by surprise at how young he looked. If I hadn't known that he was already a qualified doctor I might have thought he was 18. I felt as if I had opened the door to a sixth former whose eyes lit up the hallway with their frank intelligence. Even as I mouthed the words, I knew how irritating they must sound, but I had a compulsion to make the comment. I needed to hear confirmation that this person, who was standing in front of me, looking like the boy his father must once have been, a breed of sparrow-hawk intelligence was already a qualified doctor.

I began by asking Cosmo whether he had always wanted to be a doctor like his father.

No, not strong thoughts, not until I was eight or nine maybe, but after that I moved away from the idea. I don't know why – or whether it was just that childhood thing – all children either want to be a policeman, a fireman or a doctor, or what's the fourth thing, yeah, a spaceman. [I MANAGED TO REFRAIN FROM SAYING PERHAPS ALL BOYS DO] Or, whether it was because I always lived in a medical practice. Maybe. I was only six when we moved into a house in Notting Hill and later in Victoria that housed Dad's medical practice. I remember how on Saturdays we used to go on home visits together and how much I liked that. I would sit in his car, but with some of the older patients he would also take me on the house visits, to talk to the old people.

Saturdays were something you looked forward to, being alone with your dad?

I presume so, or it might just have been convenient for child-care because it was Saturday and Mum was still asleep and Dad was always up early because he was a doctor. Maybe it was a way of looking after me. I would wake up early because I was a child so it just made sense. Anyway, I liked it. Dad used to drive a 1970s blue Porsche – we still have the car – and I can vividly remember sitting in it and he had a car phone which looked like a brief case, very heavy and with a separate handset. I liked being in his car and looking out for traffic wardens, it was great. I remember some visits but I don't think I ever saw any children, I just remember driving around with my dad.

Do you remember any early thoughts about illness or death?

We never found anyone dead on a visit, and I don't think Dad took me to the really ill ones. I thought of doctors going to see people who had temperatures, I didn't think of any other problems I thought they only ever had the same sort of illnesses as I had and that Dad had to go to take their temperature. Strange, to think how it was a common thing to go into patients' homes then. For doctors actually to visit their patients I mean. It seemed to me like Dad went to see someone and they had a chat and then he suggested things and people seemed very grateful and pleased to see him. I quite liked my dad being a doctor and I think I would have told other people at school about our Saturday visits because I thought it was a good and an important thing to be and people are interested when you say your dad is a doctor. Everyone has had dealings with doctors and so they expect that there will be some interesting stories, unlike with other jobs, like law for example.

Were you aware that you had a grandfather who was still practising as a well-known consultant anaesthetist at Westminster Hospital, around the corner to your home and school?

I've no recollection of that at all as a young child; I think I knew that he was quite an important doctor. He never told me any stories, he has never talked about his work and I've never spoken to him about what he's done. He doesn't really talk to me, or anybody. I know the legend of him going to Buckingham Palace and doing an operation on the king, and for some reason they used one of the dining rooms. I don't know why anybody could have thought it was safe enough to do an operation like that outside of a hospital but it worked out well.

He never influenced your decision to become a doctor?

No. I must have been looking at what my parents did. I spent a lot of time on film sets with my mum and I did a lot of art at school. I was good at art and for a while I was considering being an art director because I liked creative thought and then it was a production designer and then an architect. My dad often talked about the problems of medicine and what was irritating him, or I'd be there when he answered a difficult phone call. He was always wary, even worried that I'd just go into it without enough thought, he was always sceptical. But then I decided that architecture was too office-based. I also realized that I didn't like the thought of a risky career with unsure career progression. I could never cope with the way my mum – she's a film producer – earns her money in fits and starts. Sometimes there's a lot of money and then there's none, and there can be a lot of work and projects but you may not be earning anything from that work, not for months and I don't like it, I've always hated the thought of anything unstable, I've always wanted stability. I think I weighed it all up, and I thought, I'm good at science and I like biology best, but I don't like laboratories. I like talking to people and I like the fact that people listen to what doctors have to say.

FIRST MEETING WITH COSMO

Did you have a longing as a kid to be listened to?

I have always hated being ignored, I find it very frustrating, and perhaps that was intrinsic to my decision because I still can't bear being ignored. A lot of the work is in the chatting to a patient, it's very important to me, the chatting; it makes a difference to people too.

Perhaps those early experiences with Dad are also at the roots of my interest in doing medicine outside of hospitals and working in ambulances. I have never wanted to be a GP but I've liked working with ambulances in a voluntary way since I was a teenager, and seeing medicine practised outside of hospitals. I have worked with the Red Cross for a long time but now I am doing voluntary shifts with the London Ambulance Service. I'm not allowed to get involved with the patients, not at all, at least not officially, due to insurance technicalities. I am there only to observe, but it is very hard not to be hands on and to restrain my impulses.

Aren't you more skilled than the paramedics?

No, not necessarily. Anyway, it's a very different skill set and most people think that if they got hit by a bus and someone said, 'Would you prefer a paramedic, or a doctor?' most people would say, 'A doctor.' But that would be an insane decision because most doctors would not have nearly as much relevant knowledge and experience as a paramedic who is managing that situation day in and day out.

Is that an example of the collective idealization of the doctor?

Yes, I think so. It is interesting isn't it? People always want a doctor, say when you are in a theatre or something, or on an aeroplane when they make an emergency announcement: 'Is there a doctor on board?' Doctors are used to hospitals, or their consulting rooms and to having a nurse and blood tests on hand, but a paramedic is used to working solo and under pressure. In a car crash – if you've got someone having a heart attack – you may find that the observing doctor, if there was to be one, doesn't need to lay a hand on the patient because the paramedic has done everything necessary to stabilize his patient, even if there are just technicians on board. You might still be helpful but a doctor won't usually be as hands on as a technician, not without a specialist training in trauma. In these kinds of emergency incidents there is always a process, a system in treating the patient and when it is happening you are only thinking about the next thing to be done. Even if I cannot intervene I can still be thinking ahead and getting kit out. You don't have to have a hand on the patient to be helpful. There is never time to feel anxious. You just go through the steps you need to resuscitate and you don't think about things like who the wounded person is, or anything. Perhaps I've got used to it.

I can only remember one time when I found it odd when I was physically treating a patient. It was when I was still a student and it was 10 am on a Monday morning in my last year at medical school. Someone was brought in by ambulance whose heart had stopped and who was only 30. He had been in hospital the night before, having taken an overdose but he must have gone home and had another drug overdose, not suicide. I was doing the chest compressions and this person underneath me was completely naked because you are trying to get the intravenous lines in, or to see where they have been wounded. There was a point during which I thought I might faint although I didn't but I felt very odd on top of his naked body, the oddest I've ever felt, but that was the only time I've been shocked… It was a real shame that a young person had possibly self inflicted their death by an accident, I don't think they meant to kill themselves, it affected me but then afterwards I was fine. I think with children it would be different. I would find that harrowing but I've not been involved with children and otherwise I'm fairly resilient.

Let's go back to your own childhood because that is when you discovered that you had the same genetic kidney disease as your mum, your aunt and your half brother, Ben. Did your kidney disease cause you to spend time in hospital as a child?

No, I only ever went to Outpatients where I had to have occasional blood tests.

Do you remember discovering that you had inherited the disease, or did your dad diagnose you?

I think it has always just been assumed that I would have it. I'm sure it is true that it was always just assumed I had the gene and there was never a precise point when I knew for sure.

Seems to be rather a big assumption…

I don't remember a point where it was shocking. I think – because Mum and her sister had it – we just assumed it was genetic, and everyone would have it and then I suppose it was probably confirmed at some point. I can't remember. Even now I'm meant to go to hospital for regular check-ups and I'm terrible at going. [THOUGHTFUL PAUSE] That is interesting isn't it?

Why is that?

I don't want to waste my time and have to go to a hospital appointment when I'm supposed to be at work and to sit and wait in Outpatients. It is not as if anything can be done, you know.

I think your dad said, or perhaps he was only teasing, that he bribed you to respond to my email by saying he would give you some of the blood pressure pills that you were out of, so you didn't have to waste time on going to your own GP.

Oh yes, I need to go and see Dad and collect those pills, I must get them, I haven't taken any for about a week.

You don't seem to have any anxiety – you don't go to hospital for your check ups and you run out of essential pills.

Oh yes, I'm definitely anxious but there is no point in going to hospital, it doesn't change anything, if you see what I mean?

No, I don't.

Well, they don't have anything to add to the equation. The consultants can't do anything. There is nothing that can be added to the facts, if you see what I mean?

No.

No, you don't?

No. Does your brother keep his appointments?

Well he has got diabetes too, so he needs to go to have his feet checked and his eyes checked, so yes he keeps his appointments. He really needs to go, so he does go more often than I do.

Do you think you are neglectful of yourself?

No, not at all, I take the pill, the blood pressure pill, but it's only theoretical that it might help, so I take it. When I do go to hospital all that happens is we talk about what I'm doing at my work and they want to take more blood tests, but it is just not very helpful, so I don't see any point in going. I do go occasionally, if you see what I mean, but it is frustrating that I have to take half a day off work. There is no real point.

Why do they still give you the appointments? Could the condition change? Do they need to follow you up regularly?

Mum's condition didn't change but then there was a slow deterioration over many years, which hasn't been helped by her having two kids. Yes, having kids must have made it a bit worse.

Are you knowledgeable about your condition?

Not hugely, but no one is, it's so rare but it is also very simple: it is just that my kidneys slightly leak protein and protein damages the kidneys over time.

Will your kidneys see you through?

No. No, they will fail and no one really knows when that will happen or whether the condition in our generation in less bad than in the one before. It is complicated because my brother Ben also has diabetes, which damages the kidneys as well. It is not related to the kidney condition, he is just very unlucky, so I cannot predict anything about my condition from observing him. He's my half-brother. But it doesn't mean I'm going to keep those hospital appointments because there is nothing the doctors can really add. No, it is not helpful, but it's just one of those conditions that they cannot do anything about, or predict. If I was diabetic they could offer some useful treatment. With mine there is no real treatment.

So, you are going to need a kidney transplant, like your mum?

Yeah, or I could go to dialysis first.

Is it that inevitable?

Nobody knows, not really, but probably with me it is because my kidney function is worse than it should be. But there is no way of knowing how long I will be okay, but I suppose I can predict from Mum who was 45.

You don't think any of this history has any part to play in your doing medicine?

Not really, no but occasionally I think if I become an Intensive Care Consultant or an anaesthetist, it will be helpful that I will know a friendly surgeon to operate on me, at the least I will get friendly care. Sometimes, I've thought about the care I would like, but it is not like extra time or money or anything like that could help me.

Was your training very different from your Dad's?

Yes, very different in lots of ways. His was split between getting a first and second Bachelor of Medicine where you spent between two to three, I can never remember how many years to begin with while you were only learning science and then only after that was completed you went on the wards. One year was at university and the other one was in a hospital. Dad was at University College London and then the Westminster Hospital, like his dad. The way it works now is universities are linked with a hospital. Imperial College is linked with NW London, etc. You apply to a medical school which runs you through your whole training and you still do most of your science at the beginning but there is a bit more intermingling. Now, you only get put into a firm for short periods and it is always in different hospitals, whereas Dad never left Westminster. I suppose the consultants there got to know him. I did nine weeks in Paediatrics in one hospital where I was on a firm and then I went to a different hospital to do Psychiatry. There are always pros and cons but I have had to get used to big and small hospitals and to experience the differences in rich and poor, successful and failing ones.

Which area most absorbed you in the training? Did you ever think about surgery? Did the brain interest you?

Oh, God no. Surgeons are a very odd breed altogether. As for Neuro-surgery, well I am just not interested in it. I'm afraid that when something has been damaged in your brain, well it's not like other parts of your body, you cannot often repair the brain, it is just bad news. No, I want to be an anaesthetist and to work in an Intensive Care Unit.

Like your grandfather, and yet you said he has not had any influence on you. You have also said that you are interested in the talking part of medicine but you don't have to do any talking when people are asleep. Do you know the joke, well, it's not a joke, it's an ironic statistic, or piece of research that when young doctors are thinking about a speciality, which road to take, those who decide to become psychiatrists are statistically known to have made their choice between Psychiatry and Anaesthetics.

That is what I think is wrong with the popular attitude as to be a good anaesthetist you do have to talk to the patient before surgery, to reassure them and then there is their family as well, and there is Intensive Care. You can still talk to someone who is very sick and explain that you are going to take them into Intensive Care. Yes, the majority in ICU are asleep but there are some patients who are not, and some need to be put to sleep before you take them to ICU and then there is all the other talking that needs to be done to the medical and nursing teams about the patients. I mean that you do get to talk to the patients before the operation and you get to know what they are like as a person, rather than just as a patient, before you put them to sleep. It may not be a long conversation and I've never had an operation but it can make a huge difference to how the person falls asleep, even wakes up. The other nice thing about anaesthetics is that you deal with one patient at a time, and you focus all your thoughts on them, and you can't be called away to another patient. Anyway, I

68

only said that I like talking to a person, but I didn't say that I like talking to them for a long time…

Most people are afraid of going to hospital because of their fear of an anaesthetic, and just as you say, of being put to sleep.

You bet. I would be terrified of having an anaesthetic. I'd hate it.

You wouldn't agree with your dad that the experience of an operation is a *rite de passage* to becoming a doctor?

Oh, I would. I heard a good story the other day from one of the anaesthetists I was working with last week, who was on the phone to her best friend. She is not senior, this friend, but a middle-grade anaesthetist, so she has done quite a lot and she had to have her appendix out as an emergency at Chelsea and Westminster Hospital. Apparently she was already in theatre when she saw that her anaesthetist was only one year her senior from Imperial Medical School and she burst out crying and tried to refuse to have the surgery, she was scared out of her mind. She only consented when they agreed to call in the consultant anaesthetist. It is interesting that many patients insist on choosing their surgeon, but then they have no idea about the anaesthetist. Funny, I would always want to choose my anaesthetist. After all they say that the anaesthetist is the person keeping you alive while there is someone else at your belly trying to kill you. Lots of people don't realize that anaesthetists are highly qualified doctors and they think that it is just a technical job.

What comes next for you?

I'm applying for jobs now.

I think your dad mentioned that you want to work in Accident and Emergency?

I don't know why he says that. He knows what I want to do; he is so funny. I definitely want to train as an anaesthetist but after that I'm not sure of the direction. Anaesthetists specialize in keeping you alive, how to keep your heart going, how to stop the pain, and no I don't want to be an A&E doctor. If somebody is very sick the first person who will be called to the Emergency Department is the anaesthetist, either to provide pain relief but also because we can take over, or support the patient's breathing for them.

I hear you using the pronoun 'we', so you are already an anaesthetist in your unconscious. You seem determined to work in the area of medicine closest to death.

Guess so, it is difficult. It is very hard to know until you do a job if you will like it, or be good at it. It is true there are a lot of people who die in ICU and you do have to act as a sort of gate-keeper; you make the decisions as to whether or not the patient will benefit from the treatment. No, I don't agree that it is the most pessimistic side of medicine as you are doing the most that can be done if you feel it is appropriate to offer it. What is nice is that you can do more than the other doctors can and in some ways you have got a whole lot of extra options to offer the patients.

FIRST MEETING WITH COSMO

There is still a lot more death to engage with.

Yes, although I do look after the elderly at the moment, so I am dealing with death there too. Although it is not that common to have young people dying in ICU, most patients are older. I haven't had much contact with children and I don't know what I would think about working with them.

Have you had to tell someone they are dying?

Yes, although I've not had to tell someone who still looks and feels healthy and then you have to give them a terminal diagnosis. That is the worst. I have not yet had someone I've had to say, 'Well, option A: "You are fine. Go snowboarding," or option B where the news is going to be very bad: "No, it is not looking at all good. No snowboarding for you."' I have never had to say that but I have had to look after several elderly people in hospital who are very sick and they know it. It is not quite so bad then. I think they can even feel quite relieved to know what the score is.

How do you choose to tell them?

Well, you find out what they already know and think, then you find out what others have already said, and then you get your head around their expectation; what they will tell you themselves. You try to find out where they have already got to in their own mind, and then maybe you tell them about their treatment and its effects. You tend to explain that their treatment isn't working as well as hoped and that the time has come when it is best to stop the treatment and begin to concentrate on making them more comfortable. Oh, the first thing you ask is how much they want to know and the responses are very different. You are legally bound to tell people as much as they want to know. Some don't want to know anything. It is true it is very difficult work but it is also satisfying. Now I'm thinking about it, I don't know why I find it satisfying, it is a bit odd, but you still feel like you are helping. There also has to be lots of talks with families about what is happening. You need to be sympathetic and patient. Yes, you do have to play a role, but that is always true isn't it? I can be very impatient in my daily life where I am often inclined to be sarcastic and jovial but that just wouldn't be helpful when you are talking to somebody about their death.

Yes you have to get on and deal with the procedures, whether or not the patient likes it, or wants you to. I think that telling someone else bad news is nothing like receiving it yourself. Receiving bad news is obviously so awful. No, it doesn't affect me hugely telling other people bad news, I sort of think, it's not me getting the bad news, it is not me who should be upset, but it is the patient who is going to be upset. I feel awful for them, but it's not me who has to take in the bad news. In some ways it makes me feel good, it makes me feel very glad it is not me, but it also makes me feel very bad for them. I don't know why it would upset me. This sounds weird doesn't it but I don't know why it would upset me. Most of all you would feel awful in those situations where you had to break bad news to the parents, wouldn't you? [LONG PAUSE] You hear about it don't you, people, doctors who also have children, they must think, 'Thank goodness mine are all right.' Do you think that I am weird?

No, not at all weird, brutally honest.

It is only a statement of truth: I am afraid of receiving the bad news but not of having to give it. Is that strange, do you think?

72

FIRST MEETING WITH COSMO

Not strange, just honest. Are there any regrets in your decision to spend your life in medicine?

I still can't think of anything else I'd want to do, really. It's great work and it is very variable and like anything sometimes you have a great day and others when it is very tiring. I never particularly want to leave home when I am on call but then it's not so bad. Yes, good days and bad but then you usually have a good day when you arrive and start to focus.

I have been thinking that perhaps the reason your dad doesn't think of you as wanting to be an anaesthetist is because it reminds him unpleasantly of *his* father. Were you aware as you grew up of your dad's standing and his reputation, as a doctor?

I wonder if some of my interest in wanting to deliver hospital-type medicine but outside of hospitals, is from watching Dad going to see people in their homes and carrying his bag and trying to sort it out. Looking back it's true that my whole environment was conducive to medicine, but even now Dad keeps a lot of things under his hat. Sometimes, I'll discover that he is chairman of all these different committees and speaking at universities and foreign conferences but I only ever find out in random ways. He never came home and said, 'I have been made chair, opened a hospice, or started a new charity.' You wouldn't know he is anybody special, even now that I'm a doctor myself, as he never talks to me about himself. I have watched how hard working he is. I still remember all the meals that he missed and still often does when I am planning to meet him. Yeah, he's always getting up at dawn, very early on that put me off general practice; put me off being a GP for good.

4
YOU HAVE TO DESERVE
A FATHER'S LOVE

Rachel is a GP who qualified in 1987 and worked in the NHS until 2008. She was Partner in two NHS practices for 14 years until her disillusionment with the bureaucracy caused her to leave and to join a private practice in central London.

I recall that your father was a brilliant and internationally respected pathologist, which must have been a frightening concept for a small child to grasp

I always knew he was a hospital doctor who wore a white coat, and I knew he did mysterious and messy things but I did not associate him with general medical practice. I also knew that I wanted to be a doctor from a very young age. Somebody once said, 'Oh, you want to be a doctor like your daddy!' and I said 'No – I want to be a doctor like Dr Osborne,' because he was our GP, who was also a family friend, as was often the case then, who was my first role model. Also he was Jewish and that resonated too as we were a fairly observant Jewish family. Dr Osborne was a huge guy in a dark suit with jet-black hair, always immaculately dressed with a proper black doctor's bag, smiling, caring and gentle, a real archetypal GP. Years later, after I qualified and was working as a Junior Doctor in Obstetrics and Gynaecology (and hating it, desperate to complete my GP training), I bought myself a beautiful soft dark brown leather 'Gladstone' doctor's bag and I know that this was all about trying to recreate that proper doctor in myself. I felt I needed that particular accoutrement, even though a rucksack was more practical, or some lightweight sturdy horrible polyester affair. I think that bag – which I treasure still – was as important to me as my stethoscope.

My father's work was totally different. It was a treat to be taken up to the Royal Marsden Hospital to visit him where he was head of the Histopathology Department. He was very high up in a centre of excellence, I didn't realise that as a child, not at all, it was just a novelty if my mother went shopping in the King's Road to go and visit his office. We were always taken there at Christmas and (this sounds patronizing – but it wasn't) my father was very keen that we went around the wards and cheered people up. I didn't know what cancer was then. I think I knew it was something very dreadful and frightening and my father would occasionally shake his head and remark sorrowfully that it was a terrible disease. He really was 'doing battle with it' and would occasionally say, in his dry way, 'It has got nothing going for it!' It is hard to believe now but he also kept histology samples in the dining room at home. In the 1960s he would often take my brother, who was then about 13, to attend Saturday operations with him as his clinical assistant, suitably gowned and providing his services for £1 an operation, but he became a barrister.

He had an office where there were hundreds of bottles containing specimens on shelves. Bone, or bits of liver or lung bobbing around in formalin, discoloured over many years. And there were mysterious things stained with H and E (haematoxylin and eosin) and racks and racks of microscope slides because that is what he did, and we had a lot of this stuff at home too. All Daddy needed to carry out his work was a microscope and his eyes. And when I would ask him, in genuine wonderment, 'How do you know that it is or is not cancer?' he would reply with genuine modesty and understatement, 'It's just pattern recognition.' Then there was what was called 'the cutting-up room', at the hospital. This was where he inspected the larger specimens sent to him straight from the operating theatre. His field of expertise was with skin, breast and lung cancer in particular. He would always know which operations were taking place and then he might receive a biopsy specimen or – far more disturbingly – an entire limb, or breast. He was meticulous in his work and treated the cutting-up room, with its potential for gore and horror, as a skilled chef might treat his kitchen, or a carpenter his workshop, where everything was tidied away and cleaned after each session. He would never expect anyone to clear up after him. This was particularly apparent when he carried out post-mortem examinations. He had an absolute respect for the body. I didn't go into the cutting up room and watch him working until I was about 17. I still remember the stench of formalin and formaldehyde and I could only stay in there for a little while because my eyes would be stinging, and then I had to run out of the room. Daddy lived in that room, and his clothes, everything was saturated with the smell of formalin to the point that when I went to medical school and I walked into the dissecting room where people were retching, I just said, 'God! It reminds me of my father.'

A really spooky thing happened after Daddy died, on the day he died, which was immensely shocking, as he dropped dead in the street of a heart attack, on his way to synagogue on a Saturday morning. Being observant Jews, his body needed to be buried quickly. I remember my brother and I driving across London to view his body, which was at the Chelsea and Westminster Hospital, and to try to make arrangements for the burial. As we were driving over the Albert Bridge, returning to Streatham, I was suddenly overcome by this really strong smell of formalin and I said to my brother, 'Can you smell that?' and he said, 'No,' and I said, 'Seriously, can't you smell formalin?' It was such a strong smell of my father. I remember thinking how typically macabre that was of him to have himself 'appearing' and being remembered as the smell of formaldehyde! That smell kept coming back to me for quite a few years. It was comforting, really.

I notice that you said 'his body' was taken to Chelsea and Westminster but you don't say 'he', or 'Daddy' was taken, so I am wondering whether unconsciously you feel that at that moment of death 'he' vanished?

I say that because I cannot bear to think that that thing was him: that body with a ripped shirt and an intravenous cannula sticking in his hand because the crew had tried to resuscitate him. Actually, the thing that wiped me out was not that – though God knows it was bad enough seeing his dead body – but when they gave us his belongings and I saw that his shirt had been ripped apart and that was the violent reality of his death. I knew, from having been involved with resuscitations, that there in the ripped shirt was the living information about his death.

Are you saying that for you as a doctor there is a distinction at the moment of death between the body and the human being?

I had not thought about this really at all, but I think when you see somebody die, which does not happen very often, but I have worked in Geriatrics and Oncology, specialties where death is a common event, and I have been present, on occasion, at the time of death, when somebody drifts peacefully away. That is quite different from a failed resuscitation, which is appalling and violent and desperate. With the former you only witness an absence of the person. What has popped into my mind is that I am a terrible hoarder of things and objects and yet the body immediately after death feels reduced to an object. I would not throw myself on a body and beg to be taken with it, like my grandmother's generation did, making death into high drama – I suppose it is partly because my father seemed so detached, being a pathologist. The presence of death and the knowledge of death were always there and it frightened me from quite a young age. He would tell me about cancer and what cancer did, but I didn't really understand it and it was not why I wanted to be a doctor. I remember him telling me that smoking just one cigarette could cause lung cancer and he certainly put me off that for life.

I liked the fact that he had his own room and a team of people in the laboratory, for whom he had a huge amount of respect, even though he could be an incredibly rude and impatient man – nobody behaves like that any more towards other members of staff – but he was actually very respectful and grateful to the technicians if they did their work well. Pathologists don't normally deal with patients directly and that, of course, is often why they become pathologists! The typical stereotype is that they are all crusty, awkward men with no interpersonal skills who want to hide behind their microscopes (literally and figuratively), and my father worked with some seriously odd people, but actually he was a very, very frustrated clinician who really enjoyed patient contact. His journey to Pathology began after he contracted TB about six months after he qualified, having taken Part 1 of his surgical exams (the FRCS). He was very ill, like all the junior doctors who went down like flies with TB in the late 1940s. One of the mainstays of treatment was to have the affected lung forcefully collapsed (to deprive the Mycobacterium which causes TB of oxygen and thereby killing it or at least preventing it from getting worse). This was a horrible and painful process but it was his only choice until streptomycin arrived in the UK, although he had already lost one lung by that time. He attended hospital for the treatment for five years, during which time he returned to work and took the Part 2 FRCS – passing it with ease – but was then advised not to continue with surgery as it was felt by his superiors that he was 'too weak' to tolerate such a physically demanding job. I know this was a lifelong disappointment for him. He was actually given a job by a Dr Moreland on his return, running the TB ward at UCH (University College Hospital). He then became the assistant to Prof. Cameron who was the Professor of Pathology. So he 're-qualified' as a pathologist! He was brilliant, bloody brilliant! He was a rare bird who was a pathologist, but also a surgeon who had the highest qualification, the FRCS, so his knowledge of the human body at a macro- and microscopic level was phenomenal.

On top of all that he was also an extremely knowledgeable comparative anatomist. This meant he also practised as a veterinary pathologist and he was Chief Pathologist for London Zoo and he looked after the Queen's horses too. I remember thinking that was phenomenal as a child. He did a big study of melanoma for his Ph.D and found that white horses, just as pale skin in humans, are susceptible to getting melanoma on their backsides so it was amusing as a child when, having taken the most fantastic holiday snaps he would then give us a slide show, occasionally forgetting to remove the medical slides from the box so there would be pictures of us all on the beach in Cornwall followed by a close up of a horse's arse. We would all scream!

I remember in his study at home he had a bottled foetus stained with haematoxylin and eosin so it was pink and purple. It must have been about 20 weeks old, bobbing up and down. He thought it was rather beautiful and sad. Damien Hirst had nothing on my father's collection. There is no way at all that you could do that today as it would be illegal. The foetus was sitting on the bookshelf at home. It terrified me to begin with, it was beautiful but it terrified me. Later on all the children wanted it and my brother had it in his room for years and then one of my sisters 'looked after it'. Then, when I started doing biology

A-level at school, I wanted it, so I had it in my room for a while. I think my brother has it now. Or, maybe it has been reunited with the Pathology Department's 'Specimen Library' at UCH. I was not afraid of it by then and I also knew, in that challenging teenage way, that it would freak people out. However, I also think the thought of why the foetus ended up suspended in a Perspex box, that is, its history, was very disturbing for me. The older I got, the more disturbed I found the whole concept of its existence.

My father was a pioneer of the 'frozen section'. This was such a familiar phrase for me when I was growing up. The surgeon would excise a lump, for example from a breast – a biopsy – uncertain whether or not it was malignant. This would be sent in a specimen box down a chute from the operating theatre straight into the pathology lab. My father would then rush to the lab and the technicians would freeze the biopsy into a wax block, stain it up and within a very short space of time he would have slides made up and would be looking at them down the microscope. As soon as he had analyzed them, he would call the surgeon and let them know the result. In this way, unnecessary, radical and mutilating (his word) surgery could be avoided if the biopsy proved the lump to be benign. It was ground breaking work and he would get really upset if he felt that a woman had had extensive surgery or a mastectomy unnecessarily. He sometimes felt that some surgeons had a rather cavalier attitude to their patients. Now, we are finding out that for many women, a mastectomy is not needed and indeed in some cases it would appear that the body can even rid itself of the cancer. Of course, deciding when the body can be left alone to fend for itself against a cancer and when the diseased tissue needs to be excised is the job of the pathologist. Look how cautious the men are with prostate cancer by contrast. It is an incredibly contentious field and the view is that men should not be put at risk by having unnecessary biopsies of their prostate whereas the previous generation of surgeons would whip the breast off at the first opportunity. I exaggerate, but there was undoubtedly an 'operate first and get the biopsy result after' attitude, which seriously troubled my father. I can only hope the surgery was done in good faith; one has to assume that otherwise it is very worrying.

Could your father be tender?

He could be, interestingly, with patients but with me oh, rarely, but sometimes. I had a miscarriage. I was thrilled to find that I was pregnant but at six weeks I started to bleed. My father happened to ring up that day and he asked how I was and I said, 'I've just had a miscarriage' and burst into tears. He was brilliant and said, 'I am so sorry, but you know what that means? It means you can get pregnant and that is really good.' He was right and within the year I was pregnant again. Oh God, what am I saying? He died when I was six weeks pregnant with my son, and so he never knew.

I remember he would give us bits of specimens to take into school – e.g. a liver fluke embedded in a lump of liver. But he did care passionately about the patients and he would even go down to the wards to get a sense of the patients. He believed that the history was all-important, it was all in the history and not just in the slide and he rammed that into my brain when I was a student. He was furious if he got a specimen saying 'breast' on the pathology request form. He wanted to know the age of the patient and where she was in her menstrual cycle and whether she was post menopausal and even where she was from. 'Which breast, please?' The lack of information drove him insane but because he was the specialists' specialist and the Royal Marsden is top of the tree, he was asked often for second and third opinions from all over the world. Sometimes, to a less experienced pathologist, there would be things that looked like cancer and then he would look down the microscope and say, 'Ah, yes this always looks like cancer but if you notice this particular configuration of cells you will know that in fact it is benign.' He could not bear patients having the suspense of waiting for their Outpatient's appointments and so he just rushed down to the wards, regardless how groggy they were from surgery to tell them. 'It is all right your lump is harmless.' They were always terribly grateful.

You have some of his enthusiasm haven't you?

Yes, but – you know – you can see why I have always felt an inferior fraud compared to him. If I had ended up being Professor of General Practice at Imperial College, or something, I might feel differently. But I like my clinically based work.

When, then, did you realize that you wanted to be a doctor as you are the only one out of five siblings aren't you?

Yes, I am and I don't remember ever wanting to be anything else. I do remember wheeling my dollies on the tea trolley 'to theatre'. I loved the whole hospital thing; the ambiance and I liked my father being a doctor. However, my childhood was hugely coloured by my own long-drawn-out and awful medical experiences. When I was two years old, it was my father who actually picked up that one of my hips stuck out, and figured it was something to do with my spine, which it was. I have a congenital idiopathic scoliosis. I don't know how bad it was to begin with but he took me to an orthopaedic surgeon who took a watch and wait approach and they hung on until I was eight when I went into hospital for the first time, to the Royal National Orthopaedic Hospital in

YOU HAVE TO DESERVE A FATHER'S LOVE

Stanmore. There were photos of me on the beach as a very young child when the back problem did not look that obvious but by the time I was eight years old, it certainly did. So I had my first operation and by that time I had a new medical role model who was my consultant, Mr Charles Manning, FRCS, who was a god to me but he really was the most outstanding individual as a person, as a doctor and as an Orthopaedic Consultant. He was fantastic and I adored him. He was very tall, very gentle, very kind, and he seemed to be really interested in me. He was not a cut-and-thrust surgeon. There were so many bully boys in Orthopaedics then and there still are, if less so, today.

I knew that I was going to see him because of my back and I had to have photographs taken, etc. (which I hated), but that is another thing. I just put my faith in him. When he dictated letters in front of my parents (usually my mother) and me, he would say things like: 'Rachel is now nine years old and enjoys swimming. She is getting along well at school and has been in the school play. However, the degree of her curvature has increased from such and such to such and such and I am going to carry out a rib release operation in March.' That bit, fortunately, I did not quite understand what the surgical process involved but I could see my mother was biting her nails. He would do these huge ward rounds with his entourage and spend a long time at the bedside chatting and admiring my tapestry (a hobby I took up at my mother's suggestion to pass the time while I was immobilized and which has remained a lifelong pleasure for me). And he made it all okay for me, despite the most painful surgery, and I am not going to go into detail but objectively it was hideous and gruesome and unbelievably painful and traumatic of course. Then, the same thing all over again when I was 12 years old, when I had an even bigger operation, which was even more gruesome. For all that, and the fact that I have still ended up with a most horrible looking back, I was not angry with him. Despite the suffering and promises that I would be 'better', to a degree the treatment did not work. I did not end up with a straight back and as the years have gone by, there have been many intensely painful sequelae – but I have never ever blamed Mr Manning, or seen him or his treatment as failing me. I knew that he was doing the best he could for me.

I think when I was much older – late teens, or early twenties – I remember thinking it was all a bloody con; I have still got scoliosis and surgery never got rid of my problem. I don't know if I talked to my father about this, but I think he said it was the best treatment that was available at the time, that medicine is not static but it is a living entity. I think they do get better results now, I think so. I had to wear this terrible contraption called a Milwaukee Brace that was the bane of my life.*

It really formed and informed the way I am. It is true that things change with time and my scoliosis was very bad, it was very aggressive and it was getting worse very quickly so I don't know what might have been achieved with surgery today. He was the best surgeon you could get. Yes, he was famous in his field and he was kind and being in the hospital was a secure place for me, a place where I trusted I was going to get better and everyone was nice to me, and kind and all that. I got into sewing a tapestry when I was 11 when I was on my back for more surgery and I was in hospital for four months. We were on our backs for seven weeks to the day, not allowed to sit up at all. That has all changed now. You are out of hospital in a fortnight. My mother came up almost every day from Streatham to Stanmore to see me but I don't remember my father coming and when he did, he would discuss the mechanical aspect of the treatment with the

---

* According to Wikipedia the Milwaukee brace, also known as a cervico-thoraco-lumbo-sacral orthosis or CTLSO, is a back brace used in the treatment of spinal curvatures (such as scoliosis or kyphosis) in children. It is a full-torso brace that extends from the pelvis to the base of the skull. It was originally designed in 1946 for postoperative care when surgery required long periods of immobilization.

ward sister and doctors, which was hideous I have to say. Christ! If somebody told me I had to go through that again tomorrow, I don't think I could, I just do not think I could, it was so horrible. I think my father used the experience to educate me in terms of the anatomy of the spine. I remember him drawing a picture of my wonky spine and what they were trying to do to straighten it out. The first operation did not work, but it was a preliminary for the next surgery. Flawed mechanics. Yes, two powerful men in my formative years. Charles Manning also had a passion for gardening, as did my father. With Mr Manning it was roses and I have this feeling he also bred cows and I have always had a huge fondness for cows myself. I think they are the most wonderful, gentle animals.

Your desire to be a doctor has never wavered?

No, and I think it was also a desire to try and put things right. I think the only time I changed my mind was when I was struggling so hard to get the A-level grades and I thought, 'I will have to change my mind' and I thought of nursing. But I knew that I didn't really want to do that, in spite of having incredibly positive role models for nurses. In Stanmore I lived so intimately with those women. They were like angels. I heard Mr Manning died during my first year at medical school. It must have been 1988, and I just howled for hours and hours. Mr Manning had had a stroke from which he recovered. However, it left him with some facial weakness and for a long time he would not see his young patients because he did not want to frighten them by his appearance. I remember feeling so sad when I heard that.

Everything has changed so much since my experience as a patient and I am afraid it is so often for the worse. The quality of nursing care has changed, and I can speak from a very informed position having been the recipient of so much care over the years. I also worked as a nursing auxiliary at the National Hospital for Nervous Diseases during my year off before starting medical school, which was not at all easy. What was so brilliant is that you go from being an awkward 18/19-year-old, not really skilled in social situations way out of your comfort zone, to someone who has to cope with highly dependent and disabled people. There was no room on the wards for shyness or my self-consciousness. I got used to being physically very hands on in that job and feeding and washing the patients. I am not being pretentious, but I still regard the process of laying on your hands as extremely important for all patients. Now, working as a doctor, I will hear patients complain, 'I was only in there for five minutes and the doctor didn't even touch me.'

As an auxiliary nurse I learnt how to prop up the pillows, prop them up properly, and I know it is a very important part of patient care. I cannot bear to see any patients in hospital with lop-sided pillows half fallen over. I know how to do that. You have to cross them over in an inverted 'V' and put one across the top horizontally. You have to be taught that. The technique of nursing care may not always be intellectually stimulating, but it is still fantastically important. So I did all the dogsbody stuff but I just loved it. That caring was so satisfying even making sure that the cup of tea was not three foot away from a patient who was recovering from brain surgery. Common sense but unless you have the sense and sensitivity to be that aware of your patients, you would not think to do that.

I think one of the great disappointments of modern nursing is that such details of care are considered beneath the intellect of someone with A-levels and a degree, so these 'jobs' are dispensed to a variety of nursing aides, who often have no interest in the patient at all and are not aware of the importance of maintaining a fluid intake, or the importance of turning a patient over in bed carefully. Interestingly, there were some very brilliant and very arrogant doctors on that neurological ward who were smirked about behind their backs. They were real 'alpha males'. I find Neurology and Neurosurgery attract a lot of those types, who consider themselves la crème de la crème, because they think they know how the brain works. When I started on the wards as a medical student I was shocked at how unskilled my peers were with regard to patient care. I really think everyone should have six months experience as a nursing auxiliary before they start studying medicine. There is no substitute for that experience, you cannot teach it, you have to live it and it is a humbling and invaluable experience.

When I started medical school, I thought I wanted to do Psychiatry but when I actually did the psychiatry rotation both as a student and as a junior psychiatry senior house officer as part of my GP training I really did not enjoy it at all. I felt so disappointed that it seemed only to be about giving drugs and not understanding the way the patients felt. I was not interested in giving people enough antipsychotics to get them to stop complaining that they were hearing the voices. 'Let them hear the voices,' I thought, maybe we need to work around them and their odd world not the other way round! However, it did make me realize then that what I was interested in was not psychiatry but psychotherapy, in its broadest sense, which is a major part of general practice.

When did you decide your speciality would be to become a GP?

Well, I was just rubbish at taking exams, always in a flap and panic, and so I did my basic qualifications and I think I sat the first part of the MRCP and I did not pass, no big surprise, and I thought I'm not doing that again. I always felt like a complete failure, compared to my father who wanted me to be a physician.

He did not give you any encouragement in your decision to become a GP?

He did eventually, when he must have realized, 'Why would I give this girl a hard time? She has not had the easiest time in the world.' Actually, he would often ask me about various medical conditions while I was working as a GP and he did find it impressive that GPs have such a broad spread of knowledge and practical skills even if we are not considered specialists. My mother did say, after he died, that he was very proud of me, which he did say to me once or twice. There was one point at medical school when I was really struggling and thought I was going to give up and he said something to me along the lines that he would understand if I did gave up and he would forgive me for that. I have lived under the shadow of his brilliance and it is difficult to shake that off, it really is. I always feel that I was a disappointment – but, in a way why care? Now, it is up to me whether I am satisfied with my professional life and the care I give to my patients. That is the only thing that matters at all.

What you saw in your father seems to have been an extraordinary passion and dedication as well as a volatile temper. I think you share the first two qualities with him.

Yes, I did see that in him, and, yes, I do care and worry about my patients a lot. I am always wishing that I were a better doctor than I am, a lot better, but general practice is very different from anything else. What would my father have been able to do if someone had come in and said that they had housing problems, or they had an argument with their brother or were depressed because they hated their job? He wouldn't know what to do with that. People come to a doctor with all sorts of problems. Things they used to talk to a priest about perhaps, or the extended family. If somebody isn't sleeping, or eating, or they are having panic attacks because life is so horrible then they are not well and that is a medical problem. Sometimes, patients come in with a whole set of complex symptoms and you have got to tease it all out and decide on a plan of action. As my father used to say, 'It is all in the history.' My father gave me this large book called *Nervousness, Indigestion and Pain* by Dr Walter Alvarez, published in 1943. It was about the interdependent nature of the mind and the bowel. So basically it was a huge tome all about irritable bowel syndrome. Sometimes he could kill you with kindness.

Oh, but that's what the latest IBS research is saying that they are discovering that the bowel is also composed of brain cells and has I think more serotonin manufactured in it than the brain.

Really? Well that is what this book was basically saying and I remember once complaining of headaches and back pain and my father commented that my pains were always worse when I had my exams. He really did know about stress and its effect on the body and he suffered with migraines himself (as do I) but could still surprise me with these psychological insights.

It is interesting that someone who has had as much concrete and repeated structural pain as you have had to live with have still ended up being interested in the psychosomatic, the vague and mysterious workings and disturbances of the mind. You do not even seem to get irritated with people who might be hypochondriacs.

Well, I do wonder why some people do the jobs they do! I remember taking one of my children to the doctor and she never once addressed a comment to my daughter. I think she was about four years old and the GP didn't even ask her permission to look in her ear. Oh, I really do not know why some people become doctors if they are not interested in communicating – especially with children. I love seeing children. I love to hear their take on their condition.

Having said that, I am no saint and I do get irritated sometimes. Oh, I forgot to mention that my father spoke French and Italian fluently, could get by in German and Spanish and was teaching himself Serbo-Croatian as he had so many Yugoslav colleagues and often travelled there. He was passionate about opera, had read everything on earth and was a highly knowledgeable and skilled gardener. I really had no hope, did I?

Since we last met I have been reading your father's obituaries and can see for myself what an extraordinary man and clinician he was. One of them mentions that all of his children had seen him perform a post-mortem while teenagers but you never mentioned that to me when we were last talking.

I remember the day I heard that I had got in to Newcastle Medical School and I rang him at work to tell him. I seem to remember that I could not speak to him directly as he was working in the mortuary and I rushed up to the Marsden to tell him in person. I went to his office, but he was not there. The friendly staff directed me to a ghastly ramshackle pre-fab outbuilding. I had never been there before and in fact, had always tried to avoid it. On this momentous occasion, it occurred to me that I now had no choice. It was only a matter of time before I would have to see a dead body or attend a post mortem. It was a rite of passage. I remember arriving at the door with the word MORTUARY engraved unequivocally on it. I expected to be ushered in to a sort of anteroom, where a receptionist would ask me to wait. I cautiously pushed open the door and to my horror (and it was 'horror'!) came face to face with my father, in the process of sawing off the top of someone's head. I can picture myself, flattening my back against the wall of the mortuary, trying to avoid looking at what he was doing. He was delighted, if surprised, to see me there. 'I've just come,' I said, 'to tell you that I have got in to Newcastle Medical School.' He looked up, his saw in hand, beaming at me, 'Wonderful news! Now come and take a look at this…it's very interesting…' and he beckoned me over to watch as he carefully retracted the deceased's scalp and finished removing the calvarium. I really cannot remember what the 'interesting thing' was, to my shame, as I was in a state of shock.

At the time I qualified, it was easier to become a GP and as the Membership of the Royal College of General Practitioners exam was not then particularly well respected as an indicator of academic prowess, I never sat it. I thought, 'Why should I risk putting myself through failure again for a qualification I do not even need?' Of course the situation has changed now and I would be forced to sit it in order to qualify as a GP. After I finished that hospital rotation I was never out of work. Nowadays, the MRCGP is essential and considered part and parcel of qualifying as a GP.

I would have stayed longer in Newcastle if my father had not become ill. To begin with I joined a wonderful practice in a deprived area of Camden called the Goodinge Practice, where I completed my GP training. At that time GPs still did their own on call duty at night and weekends. I was terrified of visiting poorly lit and crime-ridden housing estates in the middle of the night. I didn't feel at all safe – well, I wasn't safe – walking around at whatever hour with a doctor's bag. All I needed was a sign on my back saying, 'Mug me, I am carrying morphine.' It was a fantastic place to work and I learnt a lot from the devoted and inspiring staff there, especially my trainer, Dr David Davison.

When you look back on your 21 years in the NHS, what are your reflections?

I still miss my old patients because these are people who don't have any choice, unlike the patients you see in private practice. It was very rewarding work in many ways because we still had continuity of care in those days. The trouble with general practice now is that there are so many people who wake up with a sore throat, or a cold and want to see the doctor immediately. In the end, if you have to keep adding such patients to your surgery list as 'emergencies', it becomes a chore and you feel resentful. I also feel that society has changed and that people often do not have the support of older family members living nearby who can give practical advice and emotional support with simple issues. I also wonder, when I see people with emotional problems whether religious figures in the past, the rabbi or the priest for example, even as recently as the 1970s, may have played a bigger part than now. It is a funny position, being a GP because you know that you are nothing special and yet people put so much trust in you and have faith that you can make them feel better, or help them to feel better, in its broadest sense, and I so often feel a fraud because all I've done is to sit and listen. I don't have any particular skill or emotional trick which I use, I just listen – although I appreciate that this is what the patient needs most – for someone to sit and listen to them.

Are you still referring to emotional issues?

YOU HAVE TO DESERVE A FATHER'S LOVE

Yes, I am. A couple of times recently I've felt gratified and even flattered because I have had two patients come in, ostensibly for physical reasons, who then started to cry and related sad stories. Both said how much better they felt just by being listened to and that makes me feel really happy. If a patient complains, or if I have a really ropey consultation, it destroys me, it ruins my entire day, I can't think of anything else. I don't mean a serious complaint either, just a gripe to the practice manager, I feel awful.

I love the variety of general practice, the way that one minute you are seeing someone in emotional distress, or an acute anxiety disorder of some sort, and the next someone comes in with tummy ache.

Tummy ache seems to crop up often in other doctors' accounts. Doctors seem to feel it is one of the most difficult symptoms to assess.

I don't mind tummy ache although it is potentially very frightening and worrying. I am sure we all have our own worries. I hate headaches.

You hate headaches; although most tumours, as Martin tells me, don't begin with headaches. Why do you hate headaches?

Because I am so frightened of them. Missing something really serious. And I have.

You hate it when someone comes in with a headache.

I am very frightened of them.

DOCTORS DISSECTED

Do you tense up when someone announces a headache?

Yes, I immediately feel anxious. I get a lot of headaches myself; I get more and more headaches nowadays. I have very bad migraines. I had the most terrible one once when I was pregnant, with frightening neurological symptoms, everything broke up on the page like crazy paving and I couldn't focus properly, it was awful.

Mine are always with visual disturbance and the relief when it all returns to normal within an hour is huge.

I thought I was having a stroke the first time, but I have had some stonkers. At the moment I am going through a different style of headache, so I am trying not to think that I have secondaries in my brain from something, because, although I pretend I am not a hypochondriac, I am the worst. I have a whole imaginary medical history that I have drawn up for myself without actually consulting my GP, to the point that the other day I thought, 'Good God you haven't got a will drawn up and next week you could be dead. Shocking.'

You sound like me, the kind of hypochondriac for whom the last thing is to see a doctor.

Oh, I am too frightened to go to the doctor but I believe in my symptoms 100 per cent. The one thing I do is that I go to the opticians very regularly. I can't face the dentist at the moment as I am overdue and I am worried about what they will find! The optician seems much less threatening!

94

YOU HAVE TO DESERVE A FATHER'S LOVE

Do you think this is related to the fact that you had to endure so many invasive surgical interventions as a child?

Probably. As a child, going to the dentist was a hideous experience as they never used local anaesthetic and it was awful.

But how could that compare with the relentless pain you endured from surgery to your spine?

Nothing. But that whole back issue was enough; don't then make me go to the dentist as well! I think the difference was that whenever something major needed to be done to me, I was anaesthetized. The pain came after the procedure. At least I wasn't awake while they did the deed. That is not completely correct. There were several occasions when I had to endure some really agonizing procedures when I was conscious. No need to go into detail. The thing that still completely terrifies me is needles. I can honestly say that 'I feel your pain' when I need to inject a patient or take a blood sample. I am always immensely impressed if they do not flinch. I know that I am very patient with those who are frightened and I always say to them, 'Don't worry, no matter how much fuss you make, you will still be braver than me! You have to catch me with a butterfly net first!' Patients are grateful that you do not think they are 'pathetic'. I remember a young doctor telling me 'not to be a baby' when I was upset about his taking blood from me on my admission to hospital at the age of 11 or 12 for my spinal fusion. I would love to go back in time now and tear a strip off him for being so appallingly insensitive. Remember, in those days, parents were not allowed to stay with you to hold your hand. I cannot imagine leaving my child alone to cope with what I went through now. I remember there was a lovely nurse who held my hand and told me to help her to count the squirrels in the trees outside the window while the blood was taken. That helped me to get through the ordeal and it was only later that I realized there were probably no squirrels to count, that she was just being clever! The nurses at the Orthopaedic Hospital were angels. I will never forget them.

Have you always been a hypochondriac?

No, I think it was probably when I became a medical student. As a child I was too busy having real things wrong with me to worry about imagined ailments. I go through phases. I am very stoical, even bullish on other people's behalf, especially my husband's! If he complains of a pain in his chest, I say, 'Don't be ridiculous, those aren't the symptoms of a heart attack.' Meanwhile I am convincing myself that my breathlessness is lung cancer, even though I have never smoked and I am too scared to go to the bloody doctor. That thing when patients say: 'Oh, I don't like going to the doctor; you go in with one thing and come out with four other things.'

But usually they are people who don't look after themselves.

Not always. I don't think I look after myself. I sit there, the hypocrisy of it, giving patients advice. I don't have the right, I really don't. Once I even told myself that the pain I had in my back was just a muscle strain when it was in fact pneumonia and I was rushed into hospital because I was almost dying. That was dreadful, that was frightening.

I am worrying that what I have said implies that, without my personal medical history, I would be a very shitty doctor. I have had so much medical intervention over the years and I can still picture and remember the names of the doctors who were rude, off hand, didn't explain things properly, and who were dismissive of me. Now, I am sure I have been all of those things in my time. I know I have. No one is perfect. Patients have complained about me, not often, but it has happened. A typical scenario would be an essentially healthy person with a mild viral infection who is demanding antibiotics. Refusal causes offence sometimes, as if you are not validating their illness by refusing treatment. Such encounters always leave me enraged and exhausted.

On the other hand I can also think of the good doctors who have said, 'It's okay to feel that way.' I have experienced some awful pain under all sorts of circumstances so when a patient complains of pain I often feel I can really get inside what they are experiencing. You don't have to have asthma to know how to treat it but, for me, being able to draw on those painful personal experiences and the feelings I have had, is very useful and contributes to the 'Good Doctor' part of me. I remember the time on a Bank Holiday when I ended up in St Mary's Hospital with a strangulated femoral hernia. The staff was brilliant. Sometimes, I think to myself, 'Am I just an object that gets all these conditions in order to identify with my patients? Is this some funny joke that God is playing on me: "I tell you what, I think Rachel should end up in hospital with a strangulated hernia, then she will be able to spot it in one of her patients and truly empathize with their condition and suffering!"' Bizarre thought and, I hope, not sacrilegious!

You have had so many personal experiences of pain and it is such a difficult thing to communicate, or assess, what are your thoughts about it.

Gosh. I remember we were taught that pain is there for a reason, it's a warning, a hazard light, a useful thing and that would be the case if people didn't also suffer extreme pain with harmless conditions like IBS and headaches. There's no doubt that you see people with pains related to their unhappiness, to whatever degree and for whatever reason. Cancer, in fact, is often painless until it is too late. Patients come in, women with breast lumps, who are terrified. They often say, 'It's painful, doctor, and a friend of mine said that's always a good sign.' It is touching, because they are trying to convince themselves and the doctor that all is well. To a degree they are correct, as most breast lumps are harmless and painful breasts often indicate a condition called fibrodysplasia. I have also suffered from fibrodysplasia, which can be extremely painful and I have had fibroadenomas in the breast, which can be exquisitely tender but harmless. I used to joke that there had been a breast surgeon look at my top half in every city I have ever lived in. I've seen specialists at the Royal Marsden (of course), Newcastle General Hospital and St Mary's Hospital. I have had numerous needle biopsies and a 'punch biopsy'. Yes. More pain to add to the 'personal experience' list. It was a bit frightening at the time. In fact the vast majority of breast lumps are benign and you can confidently reassure patients of that. However (and sorry to harp back to my father again, but he knew an enormous amount about breast disease), when I told my father that I thought I was 'over-referring' patients to the breast clinic, he used to say that there was no such thing as a 'normal' breast lump. He said all breast lumps should be assessed and biopsied as the clinician could never be 100 per cent sure that they were harmless. I found his attitude reassuring but at the same time it frightened me with regard to my own lumps.

I suppose it is the difference between signs and symptoms. The symptoms are what the patient complains of and the signs are what the doctor discovers when they examine the patient. You can't ignore or refute the signs because they can be objectively confirmed and verified. The symptoms are subjective. They are what you complain of to the doctor.

YOU HAVE TO DESERVE A FATHER'S LOVE

The commonest bit of bad news I have to give these days is abnormal smears. It is never good news when I have to tell a young woman that they have to see a gynaecologist urgently. In fact, my father said, decades ago, before it was commonly realized that 'cancer of the cervix is going to turn out to be a sexually transmitted disease' and he was essentially correct. I remember his fury over Germaine Greer, who he felt was advocating unsafe and casual sex (he had strong views about this as you can imagine), because of her championing the oral contraceptive pill. His objection was not just for 'moral reasons', but more that he was very fearful about young women developing cervical cancer. He had a point, really, and we are now vaccinating young girls against the Human Papilloma Virus.

Having done 15 years as an NHS GP and now five years in private practice and with your father still so powerfully alive inside of you, would you go back and train as a doctor again, or are there are others things you would like to do?

There are other things I would like to do with my life, to make things, create things, with my hands. I would like to do more of that. I am no expert at all but I like making all sorts of things. When I was really unhappy in the NHS – coming up to when I resigned from my job – I thought, 'I hate this so much, I am going to stop being a doctor.' It was partly because the restrictions on NHS GPs had, and increasingly so, become so ridiculous. I was not able to practise medicine the way I wanted to and I thought practising medicine had become a box-ticking exercise, which had no art to it and the heart had completely gone out of medicine. I thought: 'If this is what being a doctor has become in the 21st century then I cannot do it any more.' I don't want to do it. I have always had a Florence Nightingale attitude to being a doctor; I still do have quite a romantic idea of how medicine should be practised. My father used to say repeatedly that medicine was part science and part art. I agree. So my frustrations with 'targets' and losing my clinical autonomy and ability to refer patients to whom I wanted, really killed my passion for my work. I had always been a staunch supporter of the NHS but I felt I could no longer practise medicine the way I felt was best within its increasingly strangling constrictions. Bureaucrats now run it with no interest in the personal or the individual. You really cannot 'measure' a lot of what we do – especially as GPs. To make us hit 'targets' is farcical and sometimes dangerous. It implies a one-size-fits-all style of medicine, which means that inevitably something that cannot be measured will be missed. I tried to think of other careers for myself but came to the conclusion that I was highly qualified to do very little.

I very reluctantly took this job in the private sector, thinking it would probably be an alien style of practising medicine for me. To my surprise and joy, it completely renewed my enthusiasm. I thought: 'This is what I love doing.' Apart from the independence and easy access to secondary care, I have more time for my patients and I can spend as much time as I want talking to them without worrying that the 'stop-smoking-advice-box' has not been ticked. I want to have time and energy to see my patients and to know that I can help them and not to keep apologizing because my hands are tied every time I want to refer them to a specialist or organize a test.

It is so sad to hear that said again and again during these interviews.

Yes, but it is the truth I am beginning to feel less guilty about my move, although I still feel bad when I picture my NHS patients.

YOU HAVE TO DESERVE A FATHER'S LOVE

Do I like being a doctor? Yes, I did like being a doctor and now that I am working in the private sector I still do all over again. Would I rather be an NHS doctor or not a doctor at all if that were my choice? [LONG PAUSE] I think I would still be a doctor but I suspect that I would become crabbier and crabbier and I would probably opt to do locum work because I couldn't stand the box-ticking, bureaucracy and paperwork of a GP partner. You despair. Yes, it is a feeling of despair.

5
A HOSPITAL SHOULD
DO THE SICK NO HARM

Caroline studied at Imperial College, London and continued on up the postgraduate hospital ladder to registrar status until she recently decided to give up anaesthetics to retrain as a GP.

I am currently in GP training and have just completed six months in general practice at a surgery in Twickenham. I am now back, as part of my training, working in hospital in Cardiology rotation. I will then have six months in Paediatrics followed by a final year in another GP practice in West London, to qualify for Membership of the Royal College of General Practitioners.

When did you first decide that you wanted to become a doctor?

For as long as I can remember; I have wanted to be a doctor ever since I was seven or eight but I cannot think of any experience that prompted that. My parents always said, 'Don't be teachers!' So, I knew I didn't want to do that. As long as I can remember I have wanted to be a doctor, but I still don't know why. I never struggled about which subjects to do at school, I just knew. It was only after I got into medical school, two or three years down the line that I thought, why did I choose this? I think once the reality hit me of the levels of work and responsibility, the level of commitment and time involved that I started to doubt my choice. I even started to think about other options.

A HOSPITAL SHOULD DO THE SICK NO HARM

Do you come from a medical family?

No, not at all, my whole family and extended family are teachers. I have a twin brother who is an engineer. We were brought up in Durham where I went to a girl's school until I was 18. I applied to two medical schools in London where Imperial College was my first choice. I wanted to go to the big city and I wanted to be far away from Mum and Dad, not that I don't love my parents dearly. I am very close to both of them and particularly my mother but I didn't want it to be too easy to retreat home, or for them to come and visit too often. Leaving my twin was really, really hard and he has stayed closer to home. It was harder than I thought. He got married in June and they are expecting a baby now.

I think you are married to a doctor.

I always said that I would not marry a doctor. When I started at Imperial they had this weird way of introducing you to your intake and one of the first lectures we ever had – there were 350 of us in the lecture theatre – the lecturer said, 'Have a look around, 50 per cent of you will marry somebody in this room.' For most of my medical school years I went out with somebody who works in politics and who was very removed from my professional life. Will, my husband was already qualified as a doctor when we met and had been sponsored through medical school by the Army. He is away in Afghanistan at the moment and yes, it is awful, it is very tough but when people say, 'It must be awful,' I always say that I knew what I was getting into when I married him; I have made my own bed, I may not like it but I chose it. This time around he will have been in Afghanistan for six and a half months. He was back in July at the time of my 30th birthday for almost two weeks.

Have you visited him in Afghanistan?

No. No. We are very lucky that he is in one of the big bases but because of the nature of it and what goes on there, it really is secret. He is doing a senior job, and the line is not secure when you are talking. Yes, there is a definite element of secrecy. Marrying Will was one of the reasons that shaped my career change from anaesthetics to general practice. I was all prepared to become a consultant anaesthetist – it is a great career choice for women – there is lots of flexibility, it's challenging intellectually and it is also hands-on and quite an autonomous job. Yes, you are given a great deal of independence and responsibility quite early on.

I enjoyed it all. I did three years of anaesthetics and Intensive Care medicine but then I met Will, and once we knew we were going to stay together, I started thinking differently about my career.

Unfortunately, I got quite ill about six months after we had met and that influenced my career change indirectly as well. I ended up going into hospital with what they thought was appendicitis. They operated but then I ended up with peritonitis.

After they had taken out your appendix?

Yes, after it had been taken out and then unfortunately I had to have a laparotomy, which is the big abdominal incision. When you consent to an operation the surgeon always says they are going to do a keyhole plus or minus a big procedure and you always think it cannot ever amount to that. I was in Chelsea and Westminster Hospital where I had been as a medical student but I wasn't then working there. The doctor who clerked me in was a friend from medical school and the surgeon, or assistant surgeon was also a friend.

A HOSPITAL SHOULD DO THE SICK NO HARM

Isn't it unusual to get peritonitis after you have had the appendix out?

Yes, it is. I mean there is still a big mystery surrounding what happened to me: was it negligence, or what was it? Was it a consequence of the first operation, or had they missed something the first time around? Really, I've never gone into it. Part of me thought afterwards, why did the second operation happen when I woke up to find I had had extensive abdominal surgery and ended up with a huge scar.

Did you have to have a re-section of your bowel?

No, very luckily just an open up and wash out but I was left with a very big scar. I wouldn't have said I was a particularly vain person but it is quite an emotional thing for a young girl to have to go through and there were so many things that went wrong when I was in hospital that I was left feeling very bitter about the whole thing. The hospital allowed me to become very unwell under their care and I think if Will had not been there the whole surgical procedure could have turned into a mortal disaster. You have mentioned that Martin Scurr has written about the importance on the doctor's psyche of the doctor becoming the patient, which resonates with my trajectory. I did become really unwell and there was a period of time when I still cannot recollect what was happening to me. I don't know if I have consciously blanked it out, but there are 24 hours that I cannot piece together, even though I wasn't in a coma.

Yes, I was allowed to become seriously ill and Will had to insist that I was seen by a doctor before being discharged after the first operation and then when he remained unconvinced, he had to insist that somebody more senior came to review me. Even after that, it was Will who again had to insist that the diagnosis was peritonitis and not postoperative pain. I think one of the junior doctors came to see me and I had a very enlarged and bloated tummy by this point. He examined me and then insisted that it was only abdominal gas left over from the first surgery. Will, being a doctor said, 'No it is not. She has all the signs of peritonitis, and you need to take immediate action now.' One of the concerns when you are a young woman being diagnosed with peritonitis is that as you have not had your children you worry about your womb and ovaries because everything inside of you is precious. Now, post minor surgery, I was in hospital with a septic abdomen. I woke up after the second surgery and I was really upset about the whole thing. A part of me was distressed to find a huge wound and I remember that I said to Will, we hadn't been together for long, but when I woke up and saw the bandages I said, 'If you don't want to be with me now because of the scar I understand.' It was my defence mechanism – pushing him away and giving him the get out clause – but he replied, 'I am the only one that is ever going to see the whole scar and I love you anyway.'

That sounds like a spontaneous 'engagement'.

Well, it certainly brought us closer together and I think the fact that I was ill and he was with me during that time did accelerate our relationship. I was bitter about the whole hospital thing and I have talked to other colleagues about this in our Professional Development groups, where we talk about things that have changed us as doctors. I use this scenario, not just as an example of the way I will now look after people myself, but it has also shaped my career. It led me to become disengaged and disillusioned with the NHS as an organization. I felt that I had given six years of my life to medical school and then five years post-training to the NHS. You give all of this time, energy and effort, you give up a lot of your life to do the job of being a doctor and then I felt that when I was ill I had been really let down by my profession.

At the time were you working as an anaesthetist?

Yes, and I was terrified of having anaesthetic because again it is that lack of control and you know about every possible thing that can go wrong. It was quite terrifying. I remember a girl from my year at medical school walked into the anaesthetic room and I had a panic attack and refused to have surgery and demanded they got a consultant anaesthetist, which is very unlike me but I was borderline hysterical. It should be a perk of the job, and it is professional courtesy.

This insensitive behaviour of the surgical team is awful to listen to. [Only now after editing Cosmo's interview do I realize the extraordinary co-incidence that has occurred and that Caroline is the same petrified young woman protesting about her surgery that Cosmo referred to in his interview.]

Yes, I felt that I had been really let down, that is the word and I felt that I now had the negligence as a reason to make me change direction. I thought, I have got to do something about this, and then I had the idea of becoming a GP.

Does that mean you would consider working in private medicine when you are qualified, or is your intention to become an NHS Partner?

It very much depends on Will's career. It depends on how long he spends with the Army and to where he is moved. I never know what the Army is going to do and that is a constant source of frustration to me. Whether I want to become a Partner is one of the questions that I am frequently asked in our GP training group, where I look around but nobody puts up their hand these days. I think it is 90 per cent women training as GPs now and they have chosen it because they want the working-hours flexibility. What they absolutely do not want is all the bureaucratic responsibility that goes with a partnership these days. There is also so much financial responsibility. There have been so many changes in medicine. The intake of trainee GPs in my first year at Imperial was 80 to 20 in favour of females and this year's intake, which has just joined us, is entirely women!

It's evident that you are a naturally independent person both in your choice of anaesthetics as a specialty and being able to tolerate such long periods of separation from Will. At the same time your independence is taken away by this other organization the Army. Do you have the fantasy of you and Will eventually working together?

Sometimes, I think about a little rural practice. We both want to work part-time so we can have more time together when we have children. Working together, living together, I think that might put too big a burden on our relationship and yet it could work because we work very well together as a team.

I have found that training to be a GP gives me more flexibility in terms of shift work and it is a shorter training scheme and fits in well into having to travel around the country and our geography. It will allow me to be with Will and the most important thing in my future life will be to have a family. I want to bring up my children, as we don't want a nanny. I don't want the NHS to have control over my private life, or over my future family's life.

A HOSPITAL SHOULD DO THE SICK NO HARM

I would never think of my years in anaesthetics as a waste; it was great experience looking after people who required complex management and who were often very sick.

Did you reach Registrar status?

I did two years as a Senior House Officer and then – as I had already decided to switch to general practice – I was employed as a Clinical Fellow, which has Registrar equivalence.

Can we go backwards to when you arrived at medical school? I somehow don't have the feeling that you were a rebellious teenager, but neither can I imagine you having to work very hard to achieve your place.

I was pretty good. I had my moments but I wasn't rebellious. It would sound conceited to say I didn't have to work very hard; I was always fairly academic, fairly driven, I wasn't particularly studious but I always knew what needed to be done and I did it. I wasn't someone who does the bare minimum but no, I am not a perfectionist. When it comes to revision I do enough to get the results I want.

Do you have any religious feelings?

Christian faith is part of my childhood but I wouldn't say it played a role in my becoming a doctor; it is very personal to me. I think it has become, my faith has become, stronger since I have been married and as Will has had to be away more. I find the times of our separation are when I find myself going to church more and I also think more about what faith means to me when Will is away from me. Then, I do go to church and I go to the church where we were married because it gives me that personal connection. I go to the Guards' Chapel to have that connection. Do I believe in God? I think I do. I want to have that higher connection with a spiritual energy, I like to believe that there is a higher power that can control the things we cannot. I am not a daydreamer but it is important for me to believe that there is someone, somewhere, who has a little more than mortal control.

And what about those mysterious powers of anaesthetists that Cosmo has referred to and the unique ways in which they move us through consciousness to sleep and back again?

Yes, it is one of the things that medical school never prepares you for. There were very difficult times that I remember in Intensive Care when I remember having to have painful discussions with families often at night-time about turning off the life-support machine and finding it very difficult because I wasn't prepared for those life and death situations at all. When you are responsible for making the decision and you are still a young person, it is very difficult.

You must have zoomed up the ladder very young.

Yes. I remember there was a time when I was working at a hospital in Essex and a young girl came in, who six weeks after she had given birth suffered a cardiac arrest at home. She was resuscitated but she had already been 40 minutes without oxygen. We pronounced her brain stem dead and her brain also started to swell during the night as she developed 'coning' and her death became inevitable. I was the acting registrar at the time and had to speak to her husband and parents and switch off her life support. The moment will always stay with me. It was the way the nurses laid out her body and placed a rose on her chest and she had a…a…I'm sorry but it always makes me emotional when I talk about it…she had a little photo of her six-week-old baby lying on her breast. She will never leave me; premature death is one of the things medical school never can prepare you for. Having said that I don't think you could be a good doctor if you didn't get emotional about those kinds of things. Neither do I think it should get easier because it makes you a better human if you are touched by such sadness and can experience it without becoming sentimental.

I wonder if you think there may be gender issues about the expression of feelings; Cosmo and Martin clearly shield themselves with lots of psychic armour and in Cosmo's case humour.

I think there must be but then again I don't know that it is as simple as men and women because I have had male colleagues who become visibly affected. In this instance it was the fact that she was a brand new mum. Of course I get upset when old people die, but it is the young people that make it so sad. When I was having to make decisions in Intensive Care I found it easier to justify them if it was an 85-year-old chap who has had a good innings but someone in their twenties…that is different. I am trying to compare myself to Will as a doctor. Does he get emotional…probably less so and of course he has to deal with the most harrowing things in Afghanistan. He is probably less emotional about that side of things; he has never struggled in terms of post-traumatic stress. He always thinks he has to be strong for me when he is going away and he is very protective and reassuring: 'It's not at all as dangerous as everyone says it is.' Will is an incredibly strong person and he is my level-headed rock. He is one of the kindest people I have ever known. Yes, he is my rock and he has made me a better person. He can always make me laugh at myself. It sounds gushing to say that he has made me a better person but he has made me stronger.

As I mentioned before, you come across as a strong and independent person.

It was very difficult for me the first time that he had to go away but I thought that I was working full time and must keep myself busy and there are people on the front line who are in worse positions than we are, so I think myself into a better situation. It is very hard, but it would be even harder if we had children and hopefully it will only be for another few years.

We never seem to stay with the beginning of your career and medical school – were you prepared for what you found?

No, not prepared, because it was so different from going to private school where you are spoon-fed when you turn up and are told what you need to learn and what the consequences of not doing your homework will be. At medical school you suddenly have independence and you have to make your own timetables and there is nobody to tell you what you must do. Fairly early on at Imperial we had patient contact, which wasn't clinical but about communication. I couldn't believe that I had got into Imperial

A HOSPITAL SHOULD DO THE SICK NO HARM

College, that I was in London and studying in modern lecture theatres with lots of fancy video-linking. Coming from a small northern town I felt that I was now at the centre of the modern world; I felt I had made it and was surrounded by like-minded people. I was really excited for the first few years but it is hard work and compared to other students you are doing a full-time job right from your first year. I was doing what I always wanted to do but then after two or three years as I mentioned, the work became more of a burden and I suddenly thought, 'Why am I here?' I started questioning myself about all the other things I had discounted.

Did you think about doing surgery?

I did, but you are made to choose your career path far too early after you have qualified and have to apply for a post before you have any clue about what will be right for the rest of your medical life. You are only given one year to decide before you have to apply. I didn't think about surgery thoroughly because I still wasn't sure, but when I applied for my specialty I applied for both anaesthetics and surgery. I always enjoyed being in theatre, I enjoyed the banter of it, the way the surgeon and his junior chat, the interactions with the anaesthetist and the scrub staff. Obviously, it is a very serious place but I found it fascinating to observe the ways in which people cope with the stress: some people play certain kinds of music, others want a deadly silence and others chat their way through such delicate procedures. It is a microenvironment and you are privileged to be there. Not many people get to see inside of an operating theatre, or of a body come to that.

I have heard it said that many anaesthetists chose the specialty because they prefer not to have to do much talking to patients, but you don't strike me like that at all; you feel emotionally accessible.

Hmm, yes I suppose it was an odd choice in a way, but it is only when you are doing anaesthetics that you realize that you miss that side of things, or I certainly did. I was more fascinated by the science of it. Also, I really wanted to do something hands-on. You are putting people to sleep and bringing them back to life. It is quite amazing the way it works and when you start your training in Anaesthetics you discover that nobody really yet knows how many of the drugs work. Many of them were discovered experimentally and we are still using them today without a full understanding of their scientific principles, which is again fascinating. As it happened I was offered an Anaesthetic post before the surgical applications had been processed and I thought that I better take it because it is very competitive to be in London and if I waited for Surgery I might end up with nothing.

Was there an anxiety for you in bringing somebody back to life?

Yes, and there is a great skill both to putting somebody to sleep and waking them up. In my three years I never had anyone die on the table; I have never had someone not come around but if I had completed my training it would have happened, that is the nature of the job. Distressing things like that are bound to happen, and it is not that I don't find it harrowing but it has to be a learning experience and one must use it as reflective learning. Although I allow myself to be emotional I try not to dwell on the painful moments. I don't find my work a particular emotional burden and most of the time I can leave the anxiety of it behind. The only two rotations that I haven't enjoyed have been Psychiatry at Charing Cross Hospital and Paediatrics.

Oh, that's interesting as most of the GPs I have talked to seriously thought of becoming psychiatrists.

Yes. Paediatrics, because I found it very difficult to communicate with the small children. It is very hard for children to express themselves and I found it difficult when they were upset and couldn't tell me where their pain was coming from. And then you've got the parents; numerous patients and numerous emotions as it were, and I found that very difficult. In Psychiatry, again it was the patients with psychosis and personality disorder that I couldn't communicate with on a level playing field. I wanted to be able to rationalize with them and you cannot, just as you cannot with children.

I find that very interesting because in both instances it's also about imagination and yet in conversation you are so articulate and thoughtful. But I suppose imagination is a different energy and it makes me think that maybe you are not someone who uses imagination a great deal. It interests me because in some ways imagination can become a cruel and tormenting thing. In the same way as you cannot imagine psychosis perhaps the fact that you are very rational helps to protect you from dwelling on, or imagining the danger that Will must sometimes be in.

Yes, I see myself as a pragmatic person but of course I do worry a lot. I don't want my family to worry that I worry, because I have chosen to marry someone in the Forces and I always knew that it would be difficult.

Do we choose to fall in love? Somehow those words Will spoke to you when you were in hospital in such vulnerable pain and distress sounded like an involuntary engagement.

Yes, and I will never forget that moment in the midst of so much pain and anxiety. And he meant it. Actually, I do think I have quite a vivid imagination and I can over-think things but then I can box them in and move the box over to the side. I don't want anyone to be worried about me. I think Will's mum is probably the one who knows how it feels because both her sons have been in Afghanistan, although they are not an Army family. If there was anyone I was going to talk to about the raw emotions of separation and anxiety then it would be Will's mother or other Army wives. I remember one day, after I hadn't heard from him for 10 days, I came home from work and switched on my phone and there were two missed calls. It was the worst feeling in the world knowing that I had missed his call.

When you need to be able to imagine how someone is feeling, when there is no explanation or coherence to the pain, do you become more anxious?

I don't find it so much of a struggle now in GP practice but when I did Paediatrics at medical school I had absolutely no experience of children, whereas now I have become more familiar with them and I love being with children, so that frustration has gone away. It was my failure of life experience but now I feel I am quite good at communicating with children in a way they understand. I am still learning but I am not frustrated any more.

What do you feel about mental health because that is a huge part of general practice?

Yes, it is. I enjoy the aspects of mental illness where I can see that I can make a difference, which might be doing no more than talking to people, allowing them to know that you care and want them to get better. I enjoy that but I don't think I will ever find it easy to deal with psychosis.

Have you ever suffered from depression?

Interestingly, I went to see my GP a few years back before I got together with Will. I think I was finding it hard to sleep as we were coming up to exams and I was feeling sort of, just a bit overwhelmed, and the GP, who was a locum did one of those scoring tests for depression. Oh yes, it is called a PHQ-9 and then she said that I had scored a category which diagnosed me as depressed and she gave me antidepressants. I remember walking out and throwing them straight into the bin. I was annoyed to be labelled as 'depressed' when I was only emotionally exhausted but then it is such an easy label to pin on people. At the same time I have had several friends who have been depressed and one person at medical school who was diagnosed with bi-polar illness, which did make me understand how anxious people can become in general practice that a diagnosis will go into their medical records, which is what I felt too at the time.

DOCTORS DISSECTED

We have not talked a lot about death and what it felt like to be confronting it as such a young person – I think you were only 18 when you went to Imperial.

Yes, I think anyone who says they are not deeply affected the first time…well I would be quite concerned about that. Again, nobody or nothing can prepare you for that experience. I remember when I was going out with the politician, who was not very good at dealing with emotions, and coming home from medical school after somebody had died and being very upset. He didn't want to talk about the gory details, 'You chose to do it, and so you must deal with the emotions of it.' Nobody can teach you and although I am not affected so much now, I still haven't become blasé about it. I am always affected and, yes, it is hard when you are a very young person meeting death before you are 20 and when there are now so many people in our society who go through life and never see a dead body. Yes, it is a hard thing in your first weeks to go in and see a cadaver, or an already dissected body on a slab.

Two nights ago somebody died on the medical ward. It wasn't unexpected but it was fairly quick. Her daughter came in and asked me how she had died and then she ran behind the curtain and I felt I wanted to have been able to prepare her to know that the body behind those curtains was not going to look like her mum. A dead body, within minutes, looks very different to a living body. The life has immediately disappeared. Sometimes, when you are in that resuscitation scenario you cannot predict the outcome but often you will have a good feeling about whether your attempt is going to work or not because you can see that people start to look dead. Yes, the look of someone changes quite quickly. I suppose having been in general practice and not having seen anyone die for six months and now being back in hospital I am really surprised, when I see a dead body, at how different it looks. I think for people who just see death on films and things it only looks like a sleeping body, which is very different to a corpse.

Did you grow up with a family doctor whom you knew throughout your childhood?

Yes, I did and he has only just retired. I went and did some work experience with him before going to medical school.

What do you think about the demise of the family doctor?

I think it was a lovely thing to have had growing up, to have somebody who knew us. I suppose it doesn't matter so much when you are healthy children, as we were, although I had a few problems with my ears. Having the family doctor, the way I see it now is much more important to the older generation, or people who are chronically ill. Personally, it doesn't matter to me if I go to see a doctor for a simple complaint, it can be a stranger, a man or a woman, and I don't particularly care if I see the same person. If I was a diabetic or had chronic disease, or small children, then I would want to see the same person and the role of a family doctor becomes important. I love it now when people who may be younger than me bring in tiny children and I can reassure them that their baby is healthy. It is nice to be known by your patient and to be held in a position of trust.

What do you think about the way GPs are now so rationed by time?

Where do I start with time? Simply that it is one of the biggest frustrations to any GPs work satisfaction. I was lucky that in my training practice, where I was one of the juniors, I started with half an hour but most of the partners have ten minutes and that is just no time at all; it is impossible to do a complex consultation in that time. It is not long enough to deal with emotional problems, or almost anything at all and it is a real frustration to anything except providing a simple prescription for a minor condition. When you are doing your GP training a lot of emphasis is placed on learning to listen out for a patient's hidden agenda, to what the patient does not want to talk about, and what may be going on behind the symptom. In practice we have no time at all for anything so subtle. If patients have the same doctor looking after them they can play an important systemic role which can save a lot of time by the information that you have been able to build up in the course of getting to know your patient. Particularly with older people and children, when you will already have an entire history in your head as they walk through the door. Unfortunately, that is all changing now. We do not have the luxury of time, which is very frustrating.

I have also discovered that my private life is much more important to me now than to have a high-flying career. When I was younger I was more ambitious but now I am very happy, or will be very happy, when my career plays second fiddle to my family life. I am happy for Will's medical role to be the main professional role in our family. It is funny the way it works in the Army and when I was introduced as Will's girlfriend they thought it was quite novel that I was a doctor too. They don't see many female doctors and I was called Mrs Doc, but only because I was the other half of Will. I am very happy to be called Mrs Wall rather than Dr Wall. I have changed my name professionally, but I am happy for us to be referred to as Surgeon Major and Mrs Wall. Having a family and children who are happy and that we can provide for is more important to me than a high-flying career. Historically, everything I have done has screamed 'ambition!' and yet I have never thought of myself as ambitious. Falling in love with Will has been a life-changing experience because I have found my soulmate.

6
MYSELF I MUST REMAKE

Ben has left the NHS and now works as a GP in a private West London medical practice.

I was born in the eastern side of Manchester where I was brought up in a 1930s semi-detached house; aspirational working class. My parents both left school at 14 and Mother became a secretary and Father, who was very clever, went to the local engineering company as an apprentice and trained to be a draughtsman. He attended night school at UMIST, which was then Manchester College of Technology and got his degree during the war, so quite an achievement.

Is he still alive?

No, he died aged 86 but my mother is. I suppose their aspiration was from the working class terraces to the semi-detached with the garage and the Morris Minor and in some ways their ambitions stopped there in the 1950s. They transferred their ambitions on to their children; I have an older brother. We went to the local state primary but then we were both expected to get in to Manchester Grammar School. I was a little boy from East Manchester going up to this huge and intimidating school surrounded by all the posh kids from Altrincham Prep and the ambitious Jewish boys.

Manchester Grammar was an academic factory where we took O-levels a year early so that we could all be tutored for the Oxbridge entrance exams. Nothing else mattered. It was a really impressive school with some inspirational teachers and I did all sorts of things that I would never have done otherwise, like singing requiems in Latin. My brother hated all that kind of thing. He didn't go to university, drinks beer and still goes to Manchester City football matches and he hasn't refined his voice like me. I think part of the problem was that my parents bought into the education but they didn't know how to buy into the rest of it. They thought it was too far to take us to extra choir practice or being on the touchline cheering when we played football. If I said, 'It's so cold, could you pick me up after choir?' they replied, 'No it's too late at night to drive.'

When did you decide that you wanted to become a doctor?

Well, if you had asked me at nine I would have told you I wanted to go to Egypt and be an archaeologist but at Manchester Grammar they would have said, 'Don't be silly, you must go to Oxford and study Natural Sciences, or anything that will be useful for the future.' Nothing else was acceptable and nearly everyone had to apply to Oxbridge.

Did your parents provide you with books and music at home?

There was no bookcase but there were a few books in the bottom of a display cabinet. We had a few records and an old fashioned player but there weren't anything interesting on the walls, not even mirrors. Their greatest ambition for me would have been to be a teacher as that was the next step up their social ladder and they would have understood that. When I was about 13 my grandfather died and soon after my aunt. People died unpleasantly in those days. He died without any home support and it was all down to our family who were too proud to ask for help when he got more and more ill. My mother looked after him, and I remember she was ragged from working, cooking and caring for her father. Not much time for us. It was very tense. Then her sister, who had had breast cancer nine years before, got a recurrence with a secondary lump and so my mother looked after her. Her illness was quite traumatic for me too as she had a terrible year when her lungs kept filling up with fluid. Most Saturdays I would walk to her house to keep her company and try to distract her from all the pain and play Scrabble with her and she used to say things like, 'When you grow up you'd better be a doctor so that you can cure things like this.' It was my automatic response to the helplessness I felt watching all the medical things going on in my family without any support or professional care. In my sixth form class everybody applied to medical school and some to vet school. I applied to Cambridge but didn't get in and I went to St Andrews to study Medicine.

Was that a disappointment?

I was desperate to go to Oxford or Cambridge as that was what I had been groomed for. You know the television program *Brideshead Revisited*? Well, they filmed it at Granada Studios in Manchester and they wanted some choirboys to be in one of the scenes so some of us trundled along to St Anne's Church. I hadn't read the book but I did want to watch the film and I was just blown away by this Oxbridge world; it was so romantic and I thought, 'Wow! That's where I want to belong.' I knew that I didn't fit in at home any more…and then there was the sexuality issue as well – I knew I was different to my brother – I always knew that I wasn't 'straight', my fantasies told me that.

I couldn't talk to anybody about it, it was my secret, so I was always very lonely and desperate to escape my world. I had glimpsed a world that was more exotic and which did have art on the walls where beautiful things were appreciated. I understood that we didn't have much money around, but I knew I would be swallowed up and lose myself if I didn't get away, so I went as far away as I could to St Andrews. To answer your question, I don't think it affected me that much. Perhaps that is not quite true because when I graduated from St Andrews I did go on to Magdalene College, Cambridge where I continued with Part Two and my clinical studies. It always was an ambition to be achieved. Yes, there have always been milestones to be achieved and ticked off.

Once you had got into Manchester Grammar that was the extent of your parent's support?

Yes, they could give me a desk to do my homework, but they couldn't help in other ways. They gave me the opportunity to see all these lovely things and then of course I wanted them for myself. There was this social divide and now I think I was embarrassed when they collided and I thought, 'This is just not working.' I tried to create an alternative. I didn't lie. I just didn't tell the whole truth and allowed people to assume I was from a similar background. When you are that age it is hard to make choices and know what's right; and it was then that I started to speak differently from my family. I noticed that the other kids weren't Eton posh but they spoke good South Manchester English and I adjusted the way I spoke, and later on it became Cambridge posh. So now this is my accent. St Andrews became my first escape from my family background.

It makes me think of a young cuckoo in the wrong nest.

Absolutely, but I don't think my parents had any concept of it at all; they genuinely thought everything they did for us was for the best, which it sort of was. They didn't understand anything about the experience they had dispatched me into and anyway most of it was good. Looking back now I think I did bloody well.

Medicine is an academic subject. I still feel as if I'm doing my O-levels sometimes when I come to work, but it is brilliant because it's also a job and it pays well. Am I absolutely wedded to it, like Martin? I mean if somebody said, 'Here's a million pounds to pay off your mortgage' or if I won the lottery, and somebody said, 'You can go to the British Library and restore medieval books for the rest of your life' [SAID IN A GUILTY WHISPER] I would probably do that. Something that doesn't have the weight of responsibility that is always with you being a doctor; giving people prescriptions for medications that they then take home. When I go home, I am constantly thinking, 'Gosh! I hope that person is all right.' There is always that niggle in the back of my mind and when I retire it will be a relief not to have it. If somebody messes up restoring a book then, okay, it's shocking, or if you drop the Greek urn there are still hundreds more, but no one is going to lose their life, or their child.

I find it fascinating the way you found yourself in this nest that couldn't continue to nurture you beyond early childhood. You mention that your first fantasies of sexual difference were around eight, and as Yeats said, 'Myself I have to remake,' but it is hard, not having any cultural scaffolding. I can identify with all that because there were no books in my home either, no music and I was so embarrassed if my mother spoke in Yiddish to her sister, but I was in London and everything else was on tap.

I was 18 when I arrived at St Andrews, and it's a lovely university architecturally. I met people who I never knew existed, like devout Christians, or old Etonians, there were different breeds of people that I had never come across in Manchester.

MYSELF I MUST REMAKE

You were like a duck that takes to water.

I was drunk on possibility and did everything I possibly could. I did a play in my first term. I did really well, I passed the exams and I adored doing the privileged things like anatomy dissections and learning about the physiology of the body. Perhaps I am playing that bit down, the intellectual bit, I wonder why? I did love it, and I cannot imagine my buttons would have been hit in the same way if I had done Modern Languages.

I suppose you were also meeting girls of your own age for the first time.

Yes, I was able to talk to girls, which was new. I 'came out' to the first and only person at St Andrews halfway through my first term. It was somebody who had been introduced to me as gay and I thought, 'I've got to say something,' but it took me months to build up the courage as it was the first time that I had ever mentioned sex to anybody. We did end up having an affair but I never told anybody else for the whole of that year, even though people sort of knew I was gay. It suited me to be reasonably closeted. I always thought it would be an issue being gay and being a doctor so I was very cautious. I never really came out in the hospitals, or to the consultants. It is only since being in this London practice, where I still don't come out to patients all the time, but everyone in the practice knows and I don't have to hide anything. It is just a bit of me but when you are younger it is a much bigger deal, and it can feel all consuming and is always at the back of one's mind. Now, it is only about 10 per cent of my world. Of course I am what I am because of my sexuality. I think my career might have been different if I had not been gay. As a gay man you are put in your place, even if you don't tell anyone.

You still feel that you don't quite belong; that you don't belong in the professions, or certain social areas.

Can you be more explicit?

I have had to suppress so much anger. At school I would always be called 'queer', even though I wasn't 'out', but I was always the kid in the class who does drama and sings in the choir and is not sporty, so I was called queer. I think there is something innate, as the other boys, when I look back, who were called gay, almost certainly were all gay. Yes, there was quite a lot of mental bullying at Manchester and being told you were a faggot. I think the worst insult you can find at a boy's school is to be gay, nothing worse. I always had to inhibit my emotions and play down my anger, yes to hide my emotions. I couldn't get angry, why would I get angry? You cannot respond and you can't fight back. I couldn't anyway and nobody did, so I was constantly being battered.

Were you physically small?

No, I wasn't particularly slight but I just was not sporty.

You could have given someone a punch.

No, I would certainly have come off worse, much worse, so I was constantly suppressing a very important part of my life, which affects your personality later on. I don't feel confident even now when somebody says, 'Why don't you become president of this association, or become a consultant?'

MYSELF I MUST REMAKE

What specialization might it have been with hindsight?

I don't know but it might have been Palliative Care Medicine or HIV, which is what I first came to London to do. I knew I wouldn't become Professor of Medicine, or Cardiologist, or even a surgeon. I couldn't push myself too high up the ladder because the higher you are the greater your fall. I am always aware of the fall but I don't get emotional about things, even when my father died. I was very, very upset at the time, but afterwards it was like, 'Okay and move on.' Even I thought that was a bit odd. I do get worried but I don't get emotional about my patients and I can very much compartmentalize what I do.

Earlier, you talked about the grave responsibility that is with you always.

I worry a lot about the practicalities, I worry about the margin for mistakes, or that I have hurt somebody; but even if I have to give somebody very bad news, I can still go home and have a glass of wine and watch TV, I don't get upset about it. I can control my emotions.

Are you at all sentimental?

Absolutely not. Well, hang on, maybe I have become more sentimental because I wear my father's watch, which is now really, really important to me and I also wear my grandfather's ring and that matters to me too.

I don't call that sentimental. Sentimental is crying over *Bambi* in the cinema, or not being able to think about dying children in Syria without getting teary eyed, but then doing nothing about it.

Ah, I see what you mean. Well, only recently and particularly with the Paralympics. I couldn't watch it. I would get so upset for these people who were doings such amazing things, and they would provide you with their stories, like this person who was injured in Afghanistan. It is just so tragic.

Still not sentimental in my terminology.

Well, clearly not then. No. If it is not real nothing gets at me. I was far more drawn to the Para than the Olympics proper.

If we go backwards again in time to your training what were the features that really stood out to you, that engaged you most?

Anatomy was a big thing for me, and dissecting a body is quite a privilege. There are only a few groups that are ever allowed to do that by law and full-body dissection, even in hospitals, has mainly stopped now. I thought that was just incredible and St Andrews does it over three years. You do upper limb and abdomen in the first year, chest and lower limb in the second and then brain, head and neck in the third. The London medical schools, when it was still permissible, used to do it all in one year and I am not sure you could do it justice in that time because it is a vast topic. I really enjoyed the opportunity to do anatomy in such detail. I think it harks back a little bit to my childhood when I was always the kid who would dissect the bird that had fallen off the tree;

MYSELF I MUST REMAKE

I was always curious about the insides of things. I was always squashing beetles and caterpillars and seeing what would happen if you blew them up with your cap gun, I was always using my penknife to dissect birds. I couldn't tell my parents, and if they had found out they would have thought I was really, really weird. Whenever they found out something like that, they would say, 'That's odd, it's not right, not normal, boys don't do that sort of thing.'

You were carrying a heavy Pilgrim's burden as you grew up.

Manchester in the 1970s was a pretty backward place, still facing towards another era, which was the industry of the 19th century. My parents had got their car and their china tea service for their wedding but that was where it stopped. They were very pleased to have their clock on the mantelpiece, but it was emotionally stunted and it was not acceptable for a boy to show feelings or cry at a film. There was not much love around. That sounds odd but we were not at all hugging or anything. I never saw my mother cry until her mother died. Nothing touchy feely was allowed in the family.

Were you close to your mother?

No. No, not at all. When my brother left to get married I saw her cry again. I was around 15 and she said, 'Ben, you will never leave me will you?' At that point I thought, 'I will have to leave you, in fact I will be going away as soon as I can.' And I did.

Back at St Andrews, you felt you had made the right decision for yourself?

Absolutely. The odd thing is that when you are at school and people say 'what do you want to be?' nobody tells you, 'Well, you will have at least five years at medical school.' I did seven, because I did an extra degree. It is only after you qualify that the real question arises, which is what kind of doctor do you want to be? If you decide to be a GP you now have got to do your Membership and your Diplomas of Child Health and Obstetrics and Gynaecology. It doesn't stop. I sat my last exam when I was 30-something and then I said I never want to do another. I have done far too many.

How did you end up in Cambridge at Magdalene?

Well, I must have done reasonably well. Obviously I have played myself down a bit and I did a good dissertation. I think Cambridge likes to draw people in from different environments and they always took a couple from St Andrews. Once I knew that was a vague possibility I knew that was what I wanted to do, that to study Medicine at Cambridge had to be my next step. Cambridge was like another world opening up for me. When I know what I want I am determined to get it. My aspirations now are probably not medical, they are about doing other things, or being in other places but I don't now feel any need to progress my career. Now, I am focused on progressing our practice and the business, which is very interesting. In general practice you cannot chop and change and go off and do something for two years, you have to sit there behind your desk seeing patients day in and day out, you've got to keep at it.

MYSELF I MUST REMAKE

Did you feel more comfortable in your skin when you got to Cambridge?

Yes, I did. I suppose I had created a new person. Cambridge was very interesting socially and medically. That is when I started seeing patients and travelling around hospitals. We were a very close-knit group, the medics as there were only 80 of us in the year so we got to know each other well. You have a college world and a hospital world so you also meet people who are not studying Medicine. I had friends who were Divinity students and Classicists, which is what I loved – that great broad base of learning – it is fascinating.

You were 22 then?

Yes, it was '89 when I matriculated. At Cambridge, every night there was a recital or an organ concerto going on, so much culture.

And you were hungry for it.

[GULPS] Oh, there was King's College Chapel and Trinity College Great Court. I used to go to Evensong two or three times a week. I am not religious but I just wanted to sit there and to absorb and to listen, all that beauty, that art.

What did it feel like to come face to face with a sick person after so much study, so much beauty.

It is interesting because when you have finished the theoretical part the patient is still the academic subject and then you have to relearn that these are people and vulnerable people at that. As a student clinician you are taken around by a consultant, who presents the patient to his firm as a case history. I remember the first professor I had was Professor Sir Roy Calne who was like a god of transplant surgery. Then, Baroness Warnock taught us Medical Ethics, which was extraordinary. You couldn't have made it any better, the people who wrote the best textbooks taught me. I am quite a sucker for that, I always thought this is the greatest privilege. These are Nobel Prize winners and I am going to be at the back of their ward rounds. But that doesn't mean that they are necessarily any good at communicating or dealing with people, either the patients or their students. In those days there was a sort of patient respect rather than any focus on empathy. You would go in and say, 'Hello Mrs White, do you mind if I interview you?' They might say, 'Thank you very much. Do you know you are just like my son. Pull up your chair.'

You went straight into transplant?

No, it was general surgery but there were transplants as well but you just ran around after the housemen and registrars and spent the night in theatre. I still remember the trail of ruptured bowels and stabbings and severed tendons. I suppose the next *rite de passage* was to be present at an operation, which is utterly amazing, to actually see inside somebody. These days it's all keyhole surgery or laparoscopy but then it was flesh and blood everywhere. The general surgeons were proper general surgeons – there was none of this micro-specialty – they could deal with a bowel or the liver, or kidneys. It has changed so much in 25 years. There were CT scans but only one MRI scanner somewhere up the road which was rarely used because it was so expensive. It was hands on and rather like the films of *Doctor in the House*. It was old-fashioned, you gathered by the bedside with your firm, then there would be proper medical school observations and formal teaching.

I still remember my first night in the hospital, which was probably one of the best nights – it was some bowel trauma – seeing the intestines flying out and seeing the liver and the kidneys, it was quite remarkable. Someone had been stabbed and it was a case of reconstructing the liver, which was bleeding. I was part of the on-call surgical team in Casualty. There is a huge difference between the responsibilities of a student who is watching and absorbing and being shouted at by the surgeon although ultimately you don't have any responsibility and you just do what you are told. You go away at the end of the day and don't worry whether the stitches will hold. It has to be like that because you cannot learn while you are worrying about the patient. Once you are a doctor you still have to study but you are refining the studies you have already done. I loved all the rotations and I enjoyed Paediatrics and the teamwork. Even though I was involved with a couple of dying children I didn't have the responsibility, which you do when you are the doctor in charge.

And you didn't fall in love at Cambridge?

You mean with Medicine, or a person? No, I didn't fall in love. Oh yes I did fall in love, but it wasn't requited, so that was a bit of a shame. He was one of the 'rugger buggers', who came up to me one day and confided that he was probably gay and had been in love all his life with his childhood friend...I think I had more sex at St Andrews than I did at Cambridge. The place may have been quite gay but there wasn't a lot of opportunity and there weren't gay bars, although I did go to one gay society meeting. At St Andrews the university authorities banned the gay society but that didn't seem to have any effect on the students.

There were no hiccups at Cambridge?

No, no, no, I have always done what I needed to do, what was expected, passing the exams knowing what the next steps might be, but there were no dramas, no crises, no running home, not that there was a home to run to. It was hard work but I always knew that I was going to do it.

Had you decided by now to become a GP?

No, I kept my options open. By now I had done three years at Cambridge and it was during my year at Ipswich where I felt that the hierarchy of the hospital was not conducive, well it was partly because of my concealed sexuality that I thought I wouldn't get on in Surgery.

That was a big assumption and not necessarily true.

I know that now but it was a very big part of my decision then. I never had any confusion about my sexuality, it was there from before I was five, or three or something, those were the fantasies I always had.

You don't come across at all as gay.

I think people act gay for all sorts of reasons. Some are genuinely camp and others affect it and sometimes it is part of a self-protection mechanism, or being part of a team, an outsider, or the gang, but it is a really big part of me. I knew that ultimately I wanted to share my life and world with somebody, so my quest then focused on meeting somebody I could love and live with, because being gay, the difficult thing is meeting the right person. I perceived, whether it was right or not, I perceived the hospital hierarchy of registrar, senior registrar, consultant, academic professor, or whatever, as out of my reach. I didn't feel that I would have got on in that hierarchy. I didn't feel as if I would be promoted in the same way if I also allowed myself to live the life that I wanted to live. Perhaps I was wrong. Now I realize there are lots of gay consultants around, but remember I was in East Anglia, not London which is years in advance of the provinces. Anyhow, when I was at Cambridge I didn't really know what the career options were, they didn't explain it to you; you only learn through talking to other people. Your medical education is hospital based and there is very little talked about general practice, where you need to be able to empathize with your patients. I think one of my skills, or the reason why I now do a good job, is that although I may not cry with my patients, I can empathize that this is a frightened person who feels lost in the big and unfamiliar world of disease, I can understand where my patients are and I try to look at things from other people's point of view, which a lot of doctors don't do.

Disease is a great leveller and that is what a lot of my patients find hard, they are high achieving people who are used to being in control and illness throws all that out of kilter and sometimes my patients try and keep control because disease is simply terrifying for people. I have always known how frightened people are by illness, how bewildered they are. I have seen how terrifying it is for ordinary folk. Somebody like my father would never even talk about medicine, hospital or disease, he wouldn't entertain it at all. He never went into hospital until his last illness, and in 86 years he never acknowledged having anything wrong with him. It was only in his last illness and even then he said, 'I am not going into hospital,' and I said, 'You have to go to hospital now, Dad, you have put it off this long and you've been very lucky, but you cannot ignore a bowel obstruction.' He had to have an operation and died of the consequences. If we were talking about anything medical he would leave the room, so I certainly couldn't talk to him about medicine or anything really, but I understand how hard illness is for everybody because I saw it so clearly in my own family.

After my house jobs I knew that I didn't want to continue in hospital medicine, partly because of the hierarchical structure and I thought that I would prefer to be out in the community. I moved to Canterbury and rented a flat and started at a GP practice in Whitstable. Only then I realized I didn't know a soul and was a bit lonely for a while until a friend from St Andrews contacted me, an ex in fact, and through him, I developed a group of friends in Brighton where I started to spend my weekends. I was also beginning to realize that provincial general practice was not the place to 'come out' because they are often very small communities and everybody will quickly know everything about everything. At that particular time I still was not at all comfortable with that. One of the things you get used to doing being gay is to compartmentalize your life.

I am always conscious I am meant to be talking about medical things to you and I keep talking about these peripheral things but I suppose it is because they are important to me and to my identity as a doctor. You do this kind of thing all the time, but I don't talk about myself very often. I find my train of thought going in one direction and then I think, 'I wonder if she is remotely interested in this…' You can feel very lonely when you are gay.

It is interesting that with all of these sexual abuse stories coming out people seem to forget that what I did when I was 18 was illegal and everything had to be done in secret, even though lots of men didn't have a private place to do it because their wife was around. I have learnt a lot about the gay identity and although that is not all I am, it is important to know your heritage. By my final year at Canterbury, I knew that I needed, or wanted to do something in the HIV field. There were people that I knew who had HIV and some people had died, or I knew of people who had died. It was the early 1990s and it was unimaginably terrifying. The biggest cull was in the 1990s and there was a sense of collective mourning and loss but I will want to return to that later. For my entire adult life, or adolescent to adult life, HIV had been there as a threat from the late 1980s. I went to university and there was a leaflet from the government warning us not to die from ignorance of the disease. It had always been in the background as something that was awful and threatening that might become part of me. Either I would have it, or someone I knew would have it. Then, they still advised people against testing and I didn't know whether I was HIV-positive or not, but in that situation you assume you are, you may as well be because you worry about it so much.

I remember thinking, 'So long as I can graduate here, then that will be enough, then at least my parents will be happy that I did something before I died.' It was a horrible isolation. Even at Cambridge there was always this background of underlying dread that I had made a mistake in the past that would come back to haunt or to kill me. Then there was the fact of a medical career and it wasn't clear what the recommendations were about doctors who were HIV-positive at that time. It was always a presence and perhaps that had something to do with my decision to go into general practice now I come to think of it, rather than hospital medicine, because you cannot be an HIV-positive surgeon, or a dentist. There was always this huge elephant in the room with me that I couldn't talk to anyone about. How could you confess that to your friends and anyhow at Cambridge everybody seemed straight, and there was so much prejudice and a lot of homophobia around. I don't mean it was threatening in the way it was at school but there were still jokes and comments, throwaway lines, and so I did feel – if you like – quietly persecuted. It was always at the back of my mind and I was thinking, 'If only I can qualify as a doctor at least I will have achieved something in my life before I die and then whatever happens will happen.'

It was such an important thing in my life that I thought I have got to do something, to get involved with the care of people with HIV, because if I don't do it now I will always look back and regret it and maybe I have got the empathy and skills that would be useful. I didn't know any other gay doctors, I didn't know then that London is actually full of them. I saw positions advertised for GP liaison officers at the big London centres for HIV at St Mary's and Chelsea and Westminster hospitals where there were GPs who would hold a clinic and get expertise and then liaise with the Community Care Team and the patient's GP; a perfect job for me, which I had not even known existed but I immediately knew that was the job I was suited for. I got the St Mary's Hospital job that involved working at the hospital, which had the largest HIV unit in the country and also at St John's Hospice.

I moved to London in the January of 1996 and started at St Mary's, which was another steep learning curve. In the interview – this is how naive I still was – they said, 'How do you think you would be able to help our patients with the prejudice against HIV?' I thought I was being very clever when I said, 'Well, as a gay man I think I am able to empathize with the problems and isolation the patients may have.' Now, I look back and laugh because I didn't realize that all the people interviewing me were gay and so another new world opened up.

Quite early on when I started at St Mary's and I was seeing patients with HIV for the first time and seeing what a massive impact it had on their lives – you couldn't get any more ill – and when you were prescribing for them you just thought of a dose of antibiotics and doubled it. People would die on the wards, well things were already changing, but the previous year there had been 250 deaths from HIV in the hospital, almost a death a day. At the time I started there was a research trial called the Delta Trial which was comparing single therapy to combination treatment and within the first few weeks I was there they had to halt the trial because one of the arms of the trial were dying while the other arm seemed to be recovering and they had to open the envelopes and see which method was working. The people on monotherapy were not surviving, so in that year there was a transition from people dying and being horribly ill to people being given combination therapy and surviving and it all happened within 12 months. It was remarkable that many of those people would have been dead and all those people who had already died, if only they had lived another few years, they would still be alive. There were the African immigrants who didn't have any homes or family around which meant there were a lot of legal implications, because even if somebody was in a long-term partnership and they were dying then it was still their parents who were the next of kin and would have got everything, so they had to get a will prepared. Sometimes, we would have to advise the partner to sell the house because they wouldn't be able to afford the death duties, so there were many other non-medical aspects to my work with HIV as well as dealing with all the social prejudices. It was also an amazing time because there was a lot of money around to work with. Basically the Thatcher government said, 'Don't know what to do about this; let's just pour lots of money into it and see what happens.' It filtered down right through the hospital because if the HIV department had pots of money they had to buy lots of X-ray equipment and CT scanners so the whole hospital was running on HIV money, which was its largest expenditure. I loved the work because I felt I had found somewhere I belonged and my sexuality didn't matter any more, everybody was gay so it didn't matter, my patients knew I was gay, the patients were and the consultant too. It was like chalk and cheese for me.

DOCTORS DISSECTED

You hit London at the eye of the storm when a plague seemed to have descended.

Yes, and if it hadn't been for that plague there might never have been the changes towards homosexuality in this country because it also changed medicine. Patients with HIV were often young and affluent people with influence; they may still have been leading double lives, but they knew what their rights were and there was also a big political influence from America whereby our patients were demanding to be treated with the same drugs. People now demanded first class services. We moved from a situation where nurses were sliding the food under the ward door to where the Chelsea and Westminster HIV unit had its own chef and the whole culture of the hospital, the anti-discrimination laws and equality all came about because of the way people with HIV had been treated. It also went too far the other way because people with strokes were still lingering at home. Having a stroke was not 'sexy'. No, Princess Diana didn't visit people with strokes. It was the most extraordinary and interesting time to be in the field. It is an awful disease but royalty became involved and Elton John and influential people were now coming on to the wards and huge financial donations were being made. The way people with HIV were treated became a model for the way other patients were treated. I would have half hour slots for my HIV patients, which I had never had before. Even in Oncology I had had to race through the clinics. Now I was working in a comfortable unit, which could have been in a private hospital. I was fortunate to have been part of that shared experience and, looking back on it, I think that was a good beginning for me in London, although I didn't earn very much at the hospital. There was just your basic salary as a registrar and no on-call supplements. I needed to earn some extra money so I started doing on-call for the London Lighthouse and the Griffin Project and family planning clinics. I could be seeing whole families, or sometimes people would get off the plane at Heathrow, take the Paddington Express and walk straight into the HIV unit at St Mary's from Uganda, or wherever. At the Lighthouse I got on well with everybody. That was a bizarre place looking back on it – it was like the world turned upside down for me – the entire male staff were gay, not that that is important, but oh my God it was the opposite of university.

Incidentally it was at this time that I met my partner who was working in the Hospital Liaison Team at St Mary's. We met within weeks of my arrival, so it all happened at once for me and within weeks we had decided to move in together...you just know, don't you? His previous partner of nine years had died of AIDS, undiagnosed. S had woken up to find him dead in bed, next to him, which was traumatic. S had not had an HIV test and when we started going out we assumed that he would have been HIV-positive because of the history. It happened that there was a World AIDS Conference in Vancouver later that year and S managed to go. He listened to lectures on the success of combination therapy, and how you could reduce the viral load and that life expectancy was for the first time increasing. We decided that if he was going to be tested now was the time because there was treatment available. I will never forget the day we found out he was HIV-negative. They did research on S because he should have been infected, but there are certain genetic reasons why some people are immune. At the end of that year – because for the first few months of our relationship we had had to be a little fatalistic – S realized he had a life to live and shortly after that he decided to apply to the Chelsea College of Art and become an Interior Designer. That is an important part of my story because I had always wanted to be with somebody, the whole point of everything seemed to be being a part of a partnership and for the first time in my life I was with somebody who was truly on my side.

That is what I've been saying to you throughout the interview, that you always seemed to be doing everything on your own, you went through what must have been at times an overwhelming experience, alone.

Yes, I had been looking for a partner. I don't think relationships are primarily about the lovely things like going on holiday, they are about the boring things too, like coming home from work grumpy, or how you support each other when nothing much is happening and you are not buying houses together. We have been together for nearly 17 years, so it has obviously worked and that is another incredibly important thing that I have done, or achieved. It is the most important thing in my life and if everything fell apart we would be all right. Yes, we have got all these lovely things now, we make life materially complicated but if priorities changed it wouldn't matter to me because if my relationship is there I know I will be all right.

I also knew that even though I hadn't 'come out' to my parents that eventually I would take S home to meet my family. Some time after we had moved in with each other, Mum wanted to come to London to look at some royal wedding dress, and she thought we were just flat-mates. I was 32 then but I told her that if she was coming to London she needed to understand that S and I were partners. She didn't come and both she and my father were pretty devastated. They rang me to say that I had made two old people very unhappy. They took it badly but about a week later my father rang me, he waited until Mum was out, and then he rang me to say that he still loved me. Mum never did.

Since I last met with Ben for our Christmas interview, I have heard from a mutual colleague that both he and the practice, where Ben is a partner have been deeply affected by the loss of a young and healthy male patient in his forties who had not been displaying any signs of critical respiratory illness but then died within a matter of hours and even before the ambulance could reach Intensive Care.

We begin our session informally, without any recording. While we are talking about this tragedy, about its circumstances, I notice that Ben's voice grows weaker, as if there is less air propelling him and it feels almost as if a part of him has temporarily disappeared with his memory of the untimely death.

In medicine there are very rare things that happen but when they happen to you then it is no longer rare. It is when the out of the ordinary impinges on the everyday that it makes me unnerved by life. I get through but I am always thinking – if I am walking the dog at night I look for the hooded youths ahead to avoid the confrontation if there is going to be one - I am always looking ahead to see if I can avoid the problem. I tend to be practical and pragmatic but I think it is a hard thing to get your head around when somebody the same age as you dies very suddenly and you cannot help thinking, 'There but for the grace of God go I.' It is awful and I would hate to die young like that. I kept thinking he is not going to see his children graduate, he has lost 40 years, at least, of his life and that is awful. It is a huge amount of time; it's horrible. I'm not religious so I don't think there is some great meaning to everything. I think that we are just organisms and atoms that are moved around. You can always get your head around the fact that a certain percentage of people will get cancer, or other conditions and sometimes it even happens to young people. I can process that, I can understand it and the patient has time to get used to it and their family and friends, but this was like turning a switch off. Somebody was alive and two hours later they were dead and there was nothing in between that.

DOCTORS DISSECTED

I always think it is amazing that when we go to sleep at night we wake up the next day.

When you pull back and you look at the globe with all the little ants running all over it we are so utterly insignificant but our atoms will live forever; all the iron atoms and the carbon atoms in me will still be here in billions of years, they just won't be in me but they will still be there, the energy will still be around, which I quite like. I don't need an afterlife to explain anything.

Medicine and its constant relationship to mortality are such extraordinary things. How do you find a way through the intensity of your work?

I think it is ordinary most of the time. If you are doing something day in and day out 99 per cent of it will be things you have seen before in previous consultations and even if you are dealing with extreme situations, like dying people, which is extremely emotional for all the people around, it is still something you can get used to. You have to have coping mechanisms. If you are working in a hospice you cannot become emotional about everyone who dies but you can be sad. You have to put it into context: this is the job that you are doing. You still have to function but I do think doctors can compartmentalize and put things into boxes and then move on and deal with another box with another person in it. The only way you can do it is by doing it all the time. If you were exposed to it straight away you would fall apart but the clever thing about medical school is that you are exposed to it over a period of time. First of all you are dissecting and then gradually you see people with serious problems on the ward and it will only be after five or six years that you will be asked to give somebody a terminal diagnosis, or to tell the family that something terrible has happened, although it can still be quite a young and inexperienced doctor in Casualty who has to do that. It is a *rite de passage* but you know you have done it and you will soon have to do it again because if you are a houseman in Casualty and a drowned child comes in then you will have to tell the parents. How do you get used to that? We have to remember that as doctors we are handling bodies all the time, and telling people to undress and we may have to stick our finger up someone's bottom several times a day. Sometimes we don't realize how big a deal it is for the patient lying in front of us and that what we are asking them to do is something that a patient may never have done ever before. You do have to remind yourself sometimes that some people will become very nervous in front of you.

At the end of our last meeting we finished where you had just moved to The Lighthouse as their Medical Director.

The Lighthouse was without doubt the most extraordinary and weird place that I have ever worked. It was like a Mardi Gras sort of day when the masters look after the servants and everything is turned on its head. Everybody on the staff was gay – there was just one straight person – and everything was so politically correct. You couldn't have Christmas, it had to be a Winter Festival and you couldn't judge anyone in any sort of way. When I wrote my first set of notes there was this woman who looked like a bag lady, a tramp and I put at the top 'unkempt' which was true in my opinion, looking back on it maybe it was a little judgemental, but I was reprimanded because it was her choice to look like that. The three main groups that are affected with HIV are gay white men, African men, women and children and male/female drug users and they will never get on. You couldn't find more disparate groups in society. There were also brilliant aspects to the Lighthouse. There would be open days every Friday when people came from all over the world to see the unit and talk to people with HIV. When the unit closed it joined forces with the Terence Higgins Trust but I left before it closed. I could see that my time in HIV medicine was coming to an end. If I wanted my career to progress I needed to go back into mainstream general practice. I also knew that I didn't want to go back into mainstream NHS practice in London so I applied to the Medicentres. I started off at Euston Station and ended up in Oxford Street, which was fascinating even though it wasn't challenging medicine most of the time. There was none of the satisfaction of continuity of practice that I have now, like child development.

I remember looking in the British Medical Journal and there was an advertisement in a black box, which they are usually not, which said: 'Private General Practice in West London. Please send CV.' It was a box number, all very anonymous. I sent off my letter and it turned out to be Martin Scurr's practice. This was the March of '98 and he was planning a sabbatical for 2000. I met Martin one morning when I went to see his practice and then he invited me for dinner at the Reform Club with the other doctor who worked there at the time. Have you been to the Reform Club?

Yes, once with Martin when we first met.

I had never been to one of those places before. It is quite something and we had dinner and the other doctor ignored me. Then, there was another meeting with another associate doctor and then there was a Sunday lunch that turned out to be another interview with Martin and Cosmo and a few of Martin's colleagues, and then, then he got the Human Resources Manager at Rexam PLC to interview me one evening back at the Reform Club for two hours.

MYSELF I MUST REMAKE

It was only then that Martin said, 'Okay you are the one that I want to look after my practice when I have a year's sabbatical.' This must have all been happening during '98; my selection took the best part of six months and I started working in the October. It was my first experience of the private doctor scenario.

Were you intimidated?

Yes I was, but sometimes you have to push yourself out of your comfort zone. I am not so good at it these days but then I could take a deep breath and say, 'Here is the next stage of my life, get on with it.'

Knowing about your background and how different it probably was from most of the people who were interviewing you did you ever feel that by having made that determined effort to get to Cambridge you had acquired a passport that some of these doctors might have wanted but hadn't managed to achieve? It is a grail to read Medicine at Cambridge and it surprises me how many medical applicants fail to get into Oxbridge and perhaps that allowed you to feel more confident about yourself in spite of the anxieties of not belonging to 'the club'.

Possibly. Yes, that did give me permission to push myself into something slightly out of the ordinary, I don't want to say better, but it allowed me to have professional confidence in myself. I like working at that level of excellence. I may not be the best person in our practice and I wasn't the best person at Cambridge but that doesn't matter so long as I feel I'm working to the best of my ability. Also, the style of good private medicine is exactly what every doctor would want to do: you have enough time with the patients, you have continuity of care and the satisfaction of knowing your patients, and you have the resources of London with all the private hospitals and the NHS hospitals and all the great names to refer to. When I first started at the practice it felt like being a house officer in one of the best hospitals in the world. I could ring up some top surgeon – you cannot do this in the NHS – and say, 'I have got this patient with X problem and can you now help me?' I could get an MRI scan without waiting, the patient could pay for it and there were no real restraints or frustrations. What you want to get done usually gets done without delay, whereas in the NHS you are constantly battling with the system and the funding and what you are allowed to prescribe by NICE. I don't like being told what to do either, so it gave me medical freedom to practise in the way I wanted to. It was quite daunting to begin with and I was seeing people who had known a doctor for 20-odd years and it is fair to say that they idolized Martin and then to have this young upstart sitting in his seat for a year; yes it was daunting. There was this QC who wanted to speak to Martin and he said, 'Well, he didn't tell me he was going, I couldn't do that to my clients but I will give you a go, just remember you are on trial, young man.' I could tell if I didn't come up to the mark – he would have gone elsewhere. I don't think I have ever worked as hard in my life as I did maintaining Martin's standards and going in early and finishing late, so it was a really, really, hard year sitting in Martin's chair. I was only 32 and he had nurtured this influential, high hitting, famous, and even royal clientele and he didn't want me to come in and completely scupper it and not to maintain his standards. I thought he might be going away to India for a year but he spent quite a lot of time in Norfolk. He couldn't quite let go although he did then go off to Australia for a while. I know he also had an operation and did lots of things you couldn't do if you were working and I could contact him if need be. Most of the time it paid off but I can remember one person who rang up and said, 'You didn't ring my father up after he was discharged from hospital, Martin would have done.'

Did you enjoy that year?

Enjoy...it was bloody hard work and longer hours than I would personally want to work. Martin gets up at four in the morning and I'm not made like that, but I know my limitations and that I couldn't have carried on like that, but a year is fine, because it was an important means to an end. I knew it would be a good career move to stay in the practice and I still work very hard but on my own terms.

When you were talking about your early childhood it became clear that although you parents were aspirational for you they were not able to offer you any financial, intellectual, cultural or emotional support. You had to construct yourself out of raw materials. You had to make and define yourself.

Yes, I have made myself. If you looked at me and my brother and my parents we are miles apart. If you had put me in this context all those years ago I wouldn't have fitted in, but lots of people reconstruct themselves don't they? Isn't London full of people like that?

Yes but it is hard work when you are born a cuckoo in the nest. No, you are not a cuckoo because they steal the nurture. You have had to create a symbolic sense of 'home', which we all need to thrive.

151

I didn't go home for many years because we were not welcome at home, not for a long time. My parents told S and myself that we were not welcome. I didn't go to Manchester until my father started to get ill and even then we were not welcome because an aunt and uncle still lived next door and it seemed the whole world would come tumbling down if people found out that I lived with a man in London. My parents would come and stay with us but I had not been home, or seen any of the family, for ten years. Yes, you are right, I have always been made to feel *l'étranger*, the outsider. I never fitted in. I don't quite fit in now. I take care of all these high-powered people, they are supposed to be the same sort of class as me, if you want to use a politically incorrect term, but I am not really, I have always been an outsider and I always will be. You can create yourself but you never feel real. If you have had entitlement from birth and you are helped along the way and you have been to Eton, or Winchester then you are 'there' anyway and you don't have to reconstruct yourself.

I can understand that as I've always felt an outsider too, and it doesn't matter how accomplished you become or recognized as successful and intelligent. I can never forget inside of me that I grew up in a home without any culture or secondary education and that my family started off in the rag trade in the East End.

There are still two things that I would like to hear about if you are willing, which is your time doing an MA in Art History and your son.

Jack was born in 2001. I had a friend who was a GP in Peckham who said, 'I want to have a baby.' We went out to dinner with S and at the end of the meal she said, 'I am 38 and if I haven't found the right man soon I want you to help me.' S and me said we would think about it and after some discussion, but not that much, we agreed to try and help her. It was all very amateurish and she would come over on a Sunday evening and we would do what was necessary. Artificially. By the third month she was pregnant and we were all on holiday in Elba. Jack was born in July 2001 and S and I were present at his birth, which was a very good experience. It was an interesting journey and the hospital staff were quite bemused. I am sure it is something that happens more often now.

Had you always wanted to have a child?

No, we had not discussed it as an option together until then. We told Jack's mother that we wanted to be involved in his upbringing, we are not just going to say, 'Hello and goodbye. We absolutely want to be involved in our child's upbringing too.' We tried to be involved with the pregnancy as much as we could, going to scans and things and we stayed in the house with Jack for a couple of weeks after his birth and we have been involved ever since. Jack is now 11 and we spend holidays together. S is on his birth certificate and we see each other every few weekends. He is a lovely child.

To begin with, when he was born, S would go very frequently to see Jack and I started to feel a bit left out and wanted to do something for myself. Being a bit selfish, I had always had at the back of my mind to do another qualification, some extra study in something non-medical and art based, rather than science. I did some research and found that Birkbeck College offered a Masters in Renaissance Studies. I realized that our child was going to be time consuming and that S as the biological father wanted to become more involved than me, which was fine. I didn't want to be the biological father but I did want to have something else to do when S was seeing Jack. Medicine is all consuming and sometimes it is good to think outside of the box. I was doing my day job, I didn't take any time off, Martin was back, and the University Library was open until 9 pm. I wrote essays on Titian and 'Witchcraft in German Art'. I was really impressed by Birkbeck College. Everybody was mature and committed to their subject. I got my Masters with Distinction.

What was your thesis on?

Interestingly, and I wish I hadn't now, but I went back into my comfort zone and it was on *The history and treatment of syphilis* by a surgeon called William Clowes, who was surgeon to Queen Elizabeth I. There were only three copies of this book by Clowes in existence, one of which was in the British Library, where I transcribed it for my thesis. It was amazing. The portrait of William Clowes is in the Wellcome Institute. You sit down and 20 minutes later these unbelievable manuscripts arrive and are in front of you. I was overwhelmed. If I had my life again, if I could spend my whole time looking at old books in a library or museum, or restoring old books, I would love that. I would love to be surrounded by ancient artifacts all the time.

You didn't go through a crisis – when you got a distinction – to change directions?

No, no. Well, a bit of me thought, 'Hmm, a Ph.D...' but it would have taken too long, but never say never, because the option is still there. I can do the science but there has always been the wish to address the artistic side of my personality.

MYSELF I MUST REMAKE

It seems evident to me, even if it is not to you, that if you had wanted, or perhaps if you had felt able to give yourself permission and had the confidence to pursue a clinical professorial trajectory that you have the intellectual and organizational abilities.

You have to make choices in life and it is true that when I submitted the dissertation I felt it had been too easy and perhaps I had done something wrong. Yes, perhaps if I had had more confidence in myself and in my ability and not just assumed that other people were better than me. You have to remember that when I was at my primary school I was the cleverest in my class, but when you are at Manchester Grammar you are average, or below average. At St Andrews I was a bit higher up the ranking but at Cambridge I was average again. I am always thinking, 'There is somebody else who is better than me.' I like that; it inspires me to want to better myself. I don't do envy but I am happy to be inspired by people, I know my place.

You inspire me.

It's lovely of you to say that and I am sure there are others who would say similar but when you are inside of yourself you don't feel like that. There are lots of private doctors in London and there is also a lot of ego. I think many GPs choose the private route because they cannot function in the NHS where they don't fit in. I think some of them do it for the social aspects, the credibility, and some of them because they like moving with the movers and shakers and they may 'get off' on it. I think some people like the kudos, well we all do a bit, but I don't think I am arrogant about what I do. When I meet NHS GPs at conferences they can be scathing about what I do and they don't think I am

155

really a GP. They don't think I am doing what I was trained to do, even though the actual medicine that I practise is cutting edge medicine. It makes it feel worthwhile going into work in the mornings because I haven't got a list of strangers to see. The thing that makes my job rewarding is the continuity. If you have known someone for a long time, you are even allowed to get things wrong a bit; you are allowed to say, 'Let's try this.' It might not work but at least you are doing it together with the patient and they trust you so it makes it all easier.

One of the things I find difficult and always have to remind myself because I also see people over years of their lives is that although they may feel like friends and one looks forward to seeing them every week, and I get a lot back from them as well as giving, but if something goes wrong, and I don't mean a serious ethical issue, the relationship might be over just like that.

Yes, you are only as good as your record and as a doctor I am constantly aware of that and I am always checking and then double checking, because you are giving people drugs and then they take those drugs unsupervised and who knows what could happen. I am always thinking – even though I have to take risks – that something might, or could, go wrong. For example, yesterday I had a child with stomach-ache and the question is always whether it is an appendicitis or not. If I was in the Medicentre and it was our first and possibly only meeting, I would have to say 'Go to the hospital,' but because I know the family well I could say, 'Well, he's ticking some of the boxes but not all and let's wait and see for a bit' – and if he did end up having an appendicitis I wouldn't have been wrong, it would just be that he wasn't yet showing all the signs.

MYSELF I MUST REMAKE

Talking to doctors it seems that this tiny appendage is almost the bane of their diagnostic lives, it comes up in discussion so often.

You can never predict it and every few weeks someone will come into the surgery with abdominal pain and if you get it wrong that patient could get peritonitis and die. You don't want to be over-zealous but you can never relax, it is a really hard question.

When you think about the future...

Because the most important and rewarding aspect of my life is my partnership I would not want to do anything that would jeopardize that because it is solid and central to my life. Any decision I make has to be a shared one with S. I rely on him hugely so when he goes away, like he is next week for three nights, I become really, really stressed. S would like to live abroad for a period of time. If I was going to say what I would really like to do now it would be to carry on for another ten years when I will be 55 – I have been in medicine since I was 18 – then say I have given my lot. Hopefully, I will be financially secure by then and we could go off to France. However, who knows what will happen in the next 10 years, look what has happened in the last 10. It is lovely to have that aspiration but I bet I will be working until I am 60 or more. I would hate not to have a proper retirement.

In my little, ideal world I should like to go to France and open an antique shop and make cream teas in our courtyard. That would be lovely. I would love to be pottering around antiques shops and people's houses. Yes, one day I will leave medicine behind, and it will be happily because I will have given myself fully to that career but when I close the door I won't dabble, I will close that door and say, 'That was brilliant.' I would like to feel at the end of the day I was not worrying that somebody was going to die. It is true, we go away at the weekends and I wake up in the middle of the night and think, 'I wonder how they are. How is the child with stomach-ache that I didn't send into hospital?' I worry that I don't know what has been happening to them. It would be nice not to have that worry in the back of my mind all the time.

7

IT ALL DEPENDS ON THE POINT OF VIEW

Gwen studied medicine at Cambridge and St. Bartholomew's Hospital and now works in a London NHS practice where she is non-partner.

My father came from an upper-class intellectual family who lived in Highgate and there were all sorts of people of minor importance in our family. My father is 85 now. My grandfather was a medical scientist who was part of a team of virologists which isolated influenza and he was knighted for it. His father was a microbiologist and he isolated a haemolytic streptococcus, which is what gives us our 'strep' sore throat; those were fairly significant discoveries and they were eminent men who were both at Bart's Hospital. They were reasonably well off and had a cook and a maid.

Mum comes from totally different stock – a lower-middle-class family who didn't have two pennies to scrape together. They lived in Calne where her parents worked in the sausage factory, but they also had lots of music and drama going on. My mother was the first woman in her family to go to university and she read History. Dad went to Cambridge and studied Medicine but it was difficult for him being the son of an eminent scientist and Dad became an NHS GP. Dad wasn't especially ambitious. The reason I say this is because I have been reflecting a bit on myself before our meeting; I have just attended a study group on 'burnout' and I wanted to think about why I don't think I have burned out with the stress that inevitably overwhelms all doctors in their work.

I definitely have a very good work life balance as I work three days a week which is what I have always done even before I had Joey. I am aware that I underachieve at the expense of ambition. I am a perfectionist and know that if I became a GP Partner it would put great stress on me making certain that everything was covered to my satisfaction. It would have been bizarre 20 or 30 years ago not to become Partner but things have changed since then. I was talking to my mum and she also feels she has under- achieved; she's got a brilliant mind. She reminded me that although she and my father are professionally unambitious, they have had a fulfilled and varied married life. We are a happy family, really happy although my brother was not without his problems as a teenager. We lived in a lovely house with a beautiful garden and didn't spend oodles of money on things.

When did you decide to become a doctor?

Really young; I remember thinking 'scientist' but that changed into 'doctor' quite quickly. I was the brightest in the class so there was that classic thing: the bright girls do Medicine. I was at the local girls' grammar school and there was a famous occasion when Mum responded to my exam results with, 'Only 93 per cent but what happened to the other seven?' She has no recollection of this whatsoever. I always strived to get my 100 per cent and thrived on that, and no, I didn't develop any of the accompanying eating disorders that very bright girls can suffer from. I was a little bit overweight and only recently lost that weight and I always have to watch and manage my weight but that's fine. Yes, I was really young when I decided to become a doctor but I was an all-rounder so I could have done anything but it is hard to know what my own inspiration was as I come from a family of doctors. I'm sure Dad played a part. It made sense to me because it was about doing something worthwhile as well as being intellectual and stimulating and nothing else appealed.

I used to go on home visits with my dad when he might collect me from ballet and then I'd sit in the car and wait for him. That is a strong memory. He had this enormous bell that made the telephone ring when we were in the garden so we could all hear it ring and of course I often went and sat in the surgery and waited for him. I remember those revolving note carriages and I would eat up all the biscuits and then there were the Christmas parties for doctors' children at the hospital and that kind of thing. The problem is I cannot remember ever wanting to do anything other than to be a doctor because I wanted to work with people. In fact there was a moment at Cambridge when I started to doubt it and I thought, 'What I really want is to be a social worker.'

I have never wanted to be a surgeon. I've only ever wanted to be a GP, or a psychiatrist and GPs need by necessity to have a psychological bent, but I ended up thinking general practice would be more broad, more interesting. I quite like my pharmacology and what is true about general practice is that there is never a dull moment and so much of what patients present to us turns out to be medically unexplained so that the art of medicine and the challenge of keeping the biological and the psychological in your head, as well as managing relationships and your time as well as ticking hundreds of boxes, which is what we have to do now, makes it a fast and complex process. If you see a virus or something boring you think, 'Thank God because I am horribly behind and I am slightly overwhelmed by the five depressions I've already seen this morning. So, hurrah for a sore finger.' I still get a buzz from going on my yearly 'Hot Topics' course and learning how medicine keeps moving on.

Interesting, in relation to my comment on my perfectionism, I haven't ever found general practice to be that anxiety provoking – i.e. I don't take it home and I don't worry about my patients at home in spite of being a relatively anxious and neurotic person. Although I become very anxious about other things I seem to be able to leave work at the door; even when I was training I seemed to be able to cope with uncertainty with a degree of safety netting and I still surprise myself at doing that.

Did you just sail through all the perils of being an undergraduate at Cambridge without crisis?

Erm. Do you know what? It really satisfied me getting into Cambridge I was really pleased with myself, in fact I was pretty pleased with my 10 As at GCSE and my four As at A-level. I got a buzz out of working and achieving. The problem at Cambridge was that whereas academic high achievement had been my strong suit and it was the kind of thing I could console myself with when I felt fat, or boring, or not cool enough, or whatever else it might be but when I got to Cambridge I wasn't prepared for the fact that everybody would be clever and 50 per cent of them would be brilliant as well. I wasn't prepared that they would also be slim, beautiful, trendy, worldly wise, kind and also either very sporty or incredibly good at an instrument; or all of the above. That was really hard and that was quite self-confidence bashing really.

Did you have a boyfriend?

Yes, I had had quite a few boyfriends and at the end of the first year I started going out with Luke who I went out with for three years. He was a third year and we were slightly anti-establishment and didn't go to the formal hall dinners, a bit spliff-smokey and I stopped working so hard. The first year I just scraped through although in Medicine it doesn't really matter as you just have

162

these endless hoops to pass through and you can always retake exams. I went to a May Ball and met my anatomy demonstrator who said, 'I just cannot believe you passed as you didn't do any work at all this year.' I worked quite hard in my third year and also studied Social and Political Science and I did a lot of work on Women's Studies and Gender. I also did lots of music and singing; I've done music all my life. There was lots of slightly drunken and philosophical chat – all grist to the mill. No, I didn't have a crisis and I got a good 2.1 at the end. It's interesting that you ask me about Cambridge, because ever since I came down I've been filled with regret about not getting the very most out of it, even a First, and I have a recurring dream. It is all about choosing a room in college because we had a ballot to see who got which room. I'm back in the ballot. I used to suss it out so I could get the absolutely best room in college. I still dream about the ballot and that I'm going back to Cambridge for another year to have the chance I didn't take. It is the little bit of me that wishes I had worked much, much harder. There were all these brilliant people I could have listened to lecturing and I could possibly have got a First, all these regrets even though I had such a full life.

And your relationship with Luke survived?

Yes, I went out with him the whole time and I was very in love with him actually, which was what kept me from studying more. I am not married to him; I am not married to a doctor. I am attracted to slightly controversial characters and my husband Kit is quite similar to my cousins and quite of a lot of the men in the family, but not my father, he is like the men on Mum's side. A few months after I met Kit I thought I am marrying into my family but there we go, that is what we do isn't it?

Yes, but most of us don't know that we are doing it.

In between Luke and Kit I went out with women for 10 years so I had this massive patch of lesbianism in the middle, which was slightly complicated. Yes, I left Luke for a woman who I met at medical school. I moved from Cambridge to the Royal London Hospital and Bart's and it was all very complex. She was a medic in my class. I also did an MA in Medical Anthropology at the School of Oriental and African Studies after my GP training. I wanted to be in the East End of London deliberately because I was always interested in working with the deprived. I had done my sociology and firmly had it that I was going to be an East End GP and work with the poor, which all fitted into my slightly left trajectory.

And this happened out of the blue?

Pretty much, although I knew I was bisexual so fantasy wise it was all there before. It wasn't a surprise but it was a kind of suppressed burning desire sort of thing. Complicated by the fact that it was always painful for me to have sex and which I had assumed to be psychological but it wasn't. I have since discovered that I have a physical condition, which is well described. That wasn't of course the reason I changed my sexuality but the pain confused me. I was very confused during those ten years because I was still attracted to men and got myself into situations and then had to climb out of them rather clumsily.

Was there any link between your commitment to Gender Studies and your lesbianism?

No, I knew I was bisexual but I was definitely very in love with Luke and I wasn't persuaded politically. There was just one time when I was going out with Luke when I went and did a woman's course at the Quaker's College because I was involved with the Quakers for a bit, and I kissed a girl which was pretty exciting at the time. I didn't have sex until I was 19 and then I had my dreams. I occasionally had sexual dreams that were about women, as I've said, 'Me and my dreams.' That was a clue to me but then you can also dream about having sex with all sorts of people in your life without it meaning anything. In fact Luke was unusual in his sexuality too as he was a transvestite in bed but not at any other time, which probably kept us going for quite a long time. It was perfect for him because I could desire him as a women but it didn't really work for me because he wasn't one. It really did more for him than it did for me, but hey! You are 19 and you've got time to play around with these things. He was a fascinating guy and I was really in love with him but I didn't then understand that penetration was painful not because I thought secretly that I was gay, but due to a medical condition which I could not bring myself to address until almost 10 years later. Yes, it took me 10 years to even examine myself and ask myself what is this sensitivity caused by?

It never occurred to you that your body was responsible for the pain?

No, and I didn't come across it in any of the literature while I was training and I'm very influenced by the printed page.

You were in bed with a boy dressed up as a girl and that all happened as an unconscious pairing?

Yes and, as you say, the vagaries of sexuality are so complex and variable and where – I still wonder – does the transvestite fetish come from? Luke only did it because I accepted it; he had never done it before but I already wore my bisexuality on my shoulder, from my long and frank discussions at Quaker youth camps where there were no taboos on sexual explorations.

You spent 10 years with a woman?

No, I had three relationships with women and I did have some psychotherapy at the end of that period because I was quite confused but by the time I entered therapy I had already made some decisions. I think I am genuinely bisexual and in that sense I was confused because I think you are meant to be one or the other and I am not. I did go out with two much older women, which didn't really work and they both had Chinese links as well.

I continually hear people say that if someone says they are bi-sexual they are really gay...

Absolutely, although I think people might argue that scenario more for men than women although I don't think there is any way we could be as definite and everyone is different. Having done more psychosexual medicine now, I am very aware of these differences.

It doesn't sound as though it caused you to suffer, rather more that the uncertainty was exciting.

Do you know I didn't very much, it was quite exciting and it was fun. My best friend from medical school was gay and several people who I hung around with came out of the closet and we just went around and hit the clubs for three years. It was good. I'm reasonably good at having fun and I stood on the podiums and danced the night away. The great thing about being gay is that the community is just there. It's fun and it is on the doorstep and so when I went off on my elective to Fiji we caught the bus and went off to a little gay cafe on the other side of the island. It gives you something to do and a sort of immediate identity. I was always a very 'fem' lesbian. The lesbian scene didn't really do it for me and I was much more of a fag-hag lesbian.

How did your parents respond?

Well, I had to tell them what was happening because I was living with Luke and mates from Cambridge in Archway and my brother. Then this thing happened with my new girlfriend and Luke almost had a breakdown; well he drank a lot for quite a while. I wanted to move in with her and it was fairly traumatic, now I remember it. I remember a lot of tears but it was tempered with the fact that being with her was so exciting. I felt very guilty but I also felt I had to do it.

How old where you?

I must have been about 21 or 22. I wrote my parents a letter and they wrote me a letter each by return of post. My father wrote, 'You are still my daughter and you still love medicine and music so what is the difference?' Also my grandfather of virology fame had one sister who was definitely a lesbian and used to live with a woman so it runs in the family. Mum wrote something more complicated and I remember her coming to sit on my bed when I went home and saying, 'I don't completely understand.' We had a fairly frank conversation about sex in which she gave me slightly too much information about her and Dad but she was utterly accepting. They are good at that; they are not very disapproving people. Mum is very generous of spirit and she sees the good in everybody and is endlessly and exhaustingly enthusiastic about many things. That said, I have felt her disapproval about certain things throughout my life. For example, she doesn't understand why people, particular me, would need psychotherapy. She has addressed her own unhappiness by going for a 'brisk walk', or engaging in the arts. Her side of the family is the opposite of navel-gazing. There are times when her attitude has manifest as a lack of sympathy and something of the British stiff upper lip.

Your emerging sexuality is reminiscent of a 'Spring Awakening' dramatization of sexuality.

Yes, and I'm trogging through clinical medical school at the same time. By then I was perfectly happy with jumping through academic hoops as a means to an end. I was more comfortable with being a B-grade student and I wasn't going to bust a gut to get a distinction because as far as I could tell from the doctors I was meeting it didn't make any difference in the long run in terms of your career. I was having much too much fun clubbing. I think I got the balance about right, unlike my second year exams at Cambridge when I remember not sleeping for three nights in a row.

How did you come to terms with the clinical realities of death and disease you met in London, whereas Cambridge had been limited to theoretical studies in Science?

IT ALL DEPENDS ON THE POINT OF VIEW

HIV and AIDS were big things at that time and I had a close gay friend who became HIV-positive so it was personal to me. It was a very big thing in the gay world and it was something that linked my sexuality and my medical experience with issues of stigma and medicine in a way that made sense. I had always done a lot of voluntary work and I felt I was well-placed for doing 'buddying' at Lighthouse where the training offered to volunteers was fantastic and I met more interesting people. Lighthouse gave me a good training in dealing with death and communication skills but nothing ever trains you for being a junior house officer who comes face to face with death on a daily basis as I'm sure you have already had it described.

What happens as a junior is that your bleep goes off and you turn up in the throes of things where somebody is gasping and gasping and there is a death rattle as well, but that is something else. Oh, I forgot to say that I did masses of voluntary work at the hospice in Canterbury during the sixth form, which was profound but I have only remembered it as you are guiding me through this conversation. To begin with I worked in a general hospital and mostly I was helping nurses to turn patients in their beds but occasionally I would turn up at a ward round and I think the surgeons on call used to think that I was a medical student because on a few occasions they got me to scrub up and I even assisted on an operation. It was brilliant and although I didn't want to be a surgeon the most exciting thing in the world was to stand with a retractor looking into an open abdomen. I remember famously missing my piano lesson and my mum was really cross and I said, 'But I was assisting in an operation, Mum.' Then the hospice option became more interesting to me as it was a taste of what I knew I would become because I was sitting talking to people, and I wanted to be a doctor which meant and still means to me, talking to people.

I think volunteering in a hospice might have been quite challenging to a 17-year-old.

I didn't see anybody die, but I came back and found that people had died and I remember very clearly that I blew up pink balloons in the chapel so that a dying woman could get married before she died. That is my most vivid memory of the hospice: a fact that brought home to me that people died before their time, before they were ready, before they've done everything they still want to do. I haven't had any particularly negative death experiences in my family as I don't remember the deaths of any of my grandparents being particularly traumatic. Well, that's not true, as I've just remembered my Uncle Fred's death which was very recent and that was very traumatic. Death is all still to come to me, I've got a sense of what it's going to be, but I haven't lost a parent yet and that's the hard thing. I think losing my father will be hard but he has had such an amazing life and he had this wonderful eightieth birthday with wonderful music. Now I feel he is closing his life down, although he may – like his father – go on to 92. I want him, unlike Uncle Fred, to have a good death.

What do you think about death?

[LONG PAUSE] I think I am in denial about death mostly. I am terrified of my own mortality. I've experienced relatively little bereavement and that aids and abets my denial. I think the death of your patients is emotionally relatively removed so I can deal with it plus you also have a practical role to play. I have shed tears over a couple of patients dying but it hasn't been problematic to me. The thing that I hated with hospital medicine is what it does to you because your bleep is going off! Going off! Going off! Until midnight. You don't have time to have feelings, let alone to process them because you are too busy to do anything other can cope with the practicalities of what you have to achieve with your bleep. I was 24 when I was a house officer and that meant I had much more energy than I would have now and I didn't have kids.

At that time did you think you would be permanently gay?

Yes, I did except I had had these few occasional confusing episodes with guys. I mentioned last time we were talking that going out with women didn't involve all the pain emotionally that I feel with men: will they call, won't they call? The push/pull energetic of what I feel with men, I think there must have been some fear of hurt with men and I don't know where that came from as I have left all my boyfriends and my father was incredibly present; yes a quiet but involved father. Nevertheless, I also found the whirlwind nature of men more exciting and possibly that is why I have ended up married in a heterosexual relationship. The interesting thing about Kit is that he felt different and there was something solid, certain and reliable about him and he never did that push/pull phone calls thing and he always did exactly what he said he was going to do. He was always on time for our dates. There was less of the mad excitement but there was also less of the rollercoaster painful bit and that was great.

Where did you meet?

In a bar in Brixton at 3 am in the morning, which was very funny because we both go to bed early but there was an immediate connection. I was open to the – whatever – although I was pleased to be living single for the first time in my life. In fact, when I met Kit it was a bit too soon as I was just shy of 31. I was also in psychotherapy at the time. I know I said in our first talk that I found the therapist a bit cold but that may be unfair and it did give me a sounding board.

She hasn't stayed in your mind as an internal figure?

No. No. I remember her asking at the end, 'If you were to go back into therapy would you come back and see me again?' And I said, 'Probably, because I've talked to you so much it is a bit useless starting again now.' I don't feel the need to go back into psychotherapy anyway, although funnily enough coming to see you last time was interesting because it did give me this sensation of the seduction of psychotherapy. There is this little bit of me that still wants to have the opportunity to explore it all. I quite like the praxis of everyday life and that is why medicine is so good for me and that is why going back to work tomorrow after being with the family for 11 days is good because it is so immediate and unlike sitting at your desk and doing something academic. The next moment the next patient is beside of you and you are into their world and their symptomatology. You care and you want to sort it out as best you can. It is corporeal as well as intellectual and it is so practical and of course important to the patient.

There is always so much going on in your mind at the same time, so many ideas and thought processes that you would be quite a challenge to me as a psychotherapy patient. I might have to make a decision not to listen to all the noise and ideas.

The gabble.

IT ALL DEPENDS ON THE POINT OF VIEW

Yes, the gabble. I imagine that for you being a GP and having to empty your mind, to become quiet and just focus and to listen must be relaxing; almost soothing.

That is interesting and yes it is very focused work where you are taken out of yourself and into someone else's body for a time and you need the bit of your intellect that is checking the symptoms and making a diagnosis but it is also wonderfully distracting because people are so interesting. It is true that it is rare that I am not taken inside of somebody and enthralled by their story.

As you were speaking it made me think of the role of the actor for just a moment – escaping into somebody else's body and universe.

Yes, and of course there are those very rare moments when I will be distracted, forget the lines if you like, and not be in there, but that is very rare. There are patients who make your eyes glaze over but that is different again and interesting in itself. When I sit there thinking, 'La de la, la de la I'm hearing the very same story again and again and what to do.'

I keep being struck by your passion. I know a number of GPs and work with them and for some it is just work, work done well but work and for others it is a real passion. Did you think that you would have children?

No, and when I met my Kit we decided that we were not going to have children but I changed my mind at the last minute. Initially, I thought being a lesbian wouldn't stop me getting pregnant and then I thought I didn't want to and that persisted into my marriage with Kit. At 37 I suddenly thought maybe it is a mistake not to have any children but I am only going to have the one. I have done quite well to have one but unfortunately I got post-natal depression (PND), which wasn't nice.

I got severe PND too. Once again you've taken me by surprise, as you don't immediately sound a candidate for PND. How did you understand it, as hormonal, emotional, a combination, environmental? Why do you think you developed PND? It was almost the most unbearable time of my own life.

Yes, it was horrendous and serious but only for a very short time because sertraline [an anti-depressant of the SSRI group] was brilliant and I got better on day 17. I probably recognized the onset very early but then I crashed fast and it was a very anxious depression, which would fit with my personality.

We haven't really touched on your anxieties yet have we? You seem to have such good coping strategies.

No, although anxiety often acts as a strong suit because it is a driver, isn't it? I think many GPs do have an anxious disposition which acts as a safety net because you have got so many different things going on and you have got to have a little bit of anxiety in you to make sure nothing goes wrong. You cannot allow it to become disabling but it is a useful trait for a GP.

I never took any medication and I don't know why because I had massive panic attacks and it all began when my son was handed to me in hospital and I got a blinding migraine. Did

174

yours come out of the blue? I was so shocked because with my daughter, who was our first-born, it was the most blissful year, possibly of my life.

No, there was nothing blissful about it for me. I thought it was the pits looking after a tiny baby and I had to suspend so many of my other interests. I have good family and friend relations, I belong to an intimate professional forum for personal development and I am committed to giving quality time to a small but impressive amateur chamber choir. What struck me about postnatal depression was that when I had Joey I was absolutely fine for the first three months although I always dreaded breast-feeding and retrospectively I can see that I was a little bit anxious throughout the pregnancy. I perceived having a baby as a difficult thing to do, I wanted to minimize the hardness of it and if there is anything that you cannot prepare for it is having a baby. I watched hundreds of videos on breast-feeding, but breast-feeding turned out to be fine because he co-operated well to begin with.

Which bit did you find hard, being pregnant?

No being pregnant was okay. Yes, I lost my body and I wasn't able to do that much exercise, it was a bit of a hindrance. I was fine to begin with after Joey's birth and I got into a bit of a rhythm and Kit was around too, as he freelances. I think Kit started to get postnatal depression first and then what happened was that when everything started to go wrong I tried to protect Kit by doing everything myself. He got very irritable and tired and he ended up on sertraline too but it made an enormous difference when he was able to admit that he was depressed. Joey started to refuse the breast at three months and I was completely devastated. It is one thing for me to decide to give up breast-feeding but quite another when your baby makes that decision for you and it was a disaster. I was in such a terrible state that my mother had to come straight up to London. I was in a heap and my mother came and collected me.

This is a later example of your continued perfectionism and need to be in control.

Yes, yes. Of course I was going to breast-feed for the first six months and now I was completely out of control and worst of all none of the books accounted for this. Whenever I have a problem I look for an answer and there wasn't one. My 'doctor mind' was constantly coming in to command, what is the diagnosis? I must be able to solve it. I did have the theory that his teeth were coming through very early but I also thought I should be able to get over that.

Did you ever think, 'Perhaps he doesn't like me?'

I did a little bit, well, yes I did, because it always took me ages to feed him and the other theory was that he was a big and fast-growing baby and he was just frustrated by the slowness of the breast. None of the plausible reasons I had in my mind could take away from the emotional distress I experienced when the decision was taken out of my hands. I fell apart about two weeks later when I got a massive hormone crash and so there may have been a double whammy. I also got horrific insomnia, which got worse and worse because the dopamine that is secreted when you breast-feed makes you sleepy. I got the feeling that Joey hated being a baby and I didn't like him being a baby either. The point at which I went to the GP was when I lost my appetite, that

176

was so unnatural for me, and by then I was crying all the time and inconsolable.

I felt there were insects climbing up my legs.

Yes, I had all those horrible muscle jerks and tingling.

Did that experience leave you with a lot of faith in the efficacy of anti-depressants?

Funnily enough it did, even more now. Not that I don't also have lots of scepticism about how much we use anti-depressants and how they have been marketed by the pharmaceutical companies and that people don't also have all sorts of psychological issues that they need to sort out. They bloody well did work for me and in a textbook way too. I saw a psychiatrist who told me that if you have got profound biological symptoms that is a very good marker for responding well to medication. I got better from day 17. I remember on about day 13 when I felt a brief window of improvement, the sun was out and I started singing to Joey.

Now, what I think about my postnatal depression is not only did I have the tricky baby that I couldn't control, which is my coping strategy but I wasn't going to choir, I was on leave and I wasn't going to work which gives me a strong sense of self worth, my normal relationship with my friends was interrupted and the whole baby thing also caused issues between Kit and me. I didn't feel that instant love thing for Joey but I felt the instant protection thing of wanting to get it all right. I am now madly in love with my son, literally head over heels, like falling in love, properly and it is amazing.

I didn't take anti-depressants for my postnatal depression but I did during another very anxious stage in my life, which was also characterized by rampant insomnia. I took Cipralex and it was hell on earth getting on to it; it produced suicidal ideations from nowhere, and I had to keep cutting back and cutting back the dose until I was, to begin with, only swallowing crumbs, but I am eternally grateful because I know what it can feel like and can share that with some of the patients I have who also have great difficulty getting on to medication. Some take to it like a duck to water and for others they feel as if they are poisoning themselves, to begin with.

I completely agree and I think it has totally transformed the way I am a doctor. I think I may be a bit quicker now to get out the prescription pad but to be honest with you that is because we are manacled anyway. People often only come to see me at the point of desperation and you might hold off for a week because there may be an improvement just from talking to them but the reality is that while we can offer some psychological therapy it will take three months of waiting time, so it is not much of an option. I am sure if I could be confident of saying, 'Ring this number and someone will see you next week,' it would make a huge difference to people's choice. I actually think that anti-depressants work reasonably well for the majority and when they don't there is often something else going on in their family. Although I wasn't ever like you, suicidal, I did discover that the state of depression that I was in, if it had not lifted, if I had not been assured by professionals that I would get better, my experience of it was so severe that if it was unrelieved it would not have been compatible with life. Yes, I also gained enormous insight into what it can feel like for my patients to feel suicidal. It was a complete insight into the mystery of why people would kill themselves. I have almost lost the immediacy of the sensation now, but I will always have it in the back of my mind. I didn't have any desire to kill myself because I also thought, 'I have had such a brilliant time in my life,' I could rationalize that I just had to get through every day of feeling shit and then I would get better.

I do love being a GP, there is just no question about it and I was thinking about how I may not have expressed that to you sufficiently in our last meeting. I love the combination of being drawn into somebody else's world and the practical usefulness of it because it feels so good helping people to feel better. I find my afternoon with paperwork to be so, so dull. I couldn't be an academic, and even doing my Masters, it wasn't grounded enough in the everyday. I like gardening and cooking and playing with Joey. Last week, after Joey had his minor operation on his ears we had such a special afternoon playing together.

What did it feel like last week as a doctor and a mum having to hand Joey's care over to other professionals? Was it difficult? Was Kit with you?

That is really interesting. Yes, Kit came to the hospital too; he wanted to be there. I felt like I could have done it on my own but it was great that he could be there too. Luckily, the general ward had an amazing playroom which got us through the first three hours of waiting to go into theatre and then the nurse took us to the anaesthetic room and she was blowing bubbles and Joey was so brave. The anaesthetist, who was a very gentle man said, 'There's the space mask and now we have to blow up the green balloon,' which Joey did so conscientiously: 'Whhh, whhh.' He was in my arms when he fell asleep and then the anaesthetist said, 'Would you like to give him a kiss?' He repeated the question to Kit, 'Would you like to give him a kiss?' I hadn't thought of kissing him and then I thought, 'Perhaps he is asking me to give him a kiss in case it is the last one,' which hadn't crossed my mind. As I walked out, I felt prickly teary and I'm not sure I would have otherwise.

A farewell kiss...

Exactly, a farewell kiss, and that shook me even though I had not been particularly concerned as it was such a small routine procedure. We got a sandwich and we were given a bleep to tell us when Joey was waking up but we just wanted to stand outside of the recovery room. I was glad I did that because when the bleep went off, through the thick double doors, I could hear crying and I could tell Joey was really distressed and we were both hammering on the thick double-glass doors, 'Let us in!' The busy nurses seemed to take ages coming. That kiss was the thing that got me, even more distressing than seeing him lying limp and asleep.

I know that you have already done a diploma in Psychosexual Medicine and wanted to ask you a little bit about the nature of dealing with the body in the consulting room, whether there is any eroticism for you and I don't in any sense mean sexual transgression.

I haven't thought about this in detail but there really is nothing sexual about the physical examination because it is so focused and the requirement to look at the body as part of your information gathering exercise if you like. That is purely the case if you are looking at a mole on an arm, I suppose it is different when you are doing a genital examination but even breast examinations feel routine and practical when you are so busy feeling for your

180

lump. The complexity around it is more the communication of undressing and what you are then going to do and it is interesting of course if you observe your patient's reaction to the undressing. Yes, I suppose there are moments when that eroticism does pop up. Recently, I saw a Scandinavian woman who had an itchy rash on her body and she obviously didn't wear a bra. She was very vigorous and enthusiastic and stood up in front of me and pulled her top up and there was nothing on underneath and she was showing me the rash, and everything was jiggling around with such enthusiasm. It did seem quite odd to have this blonde Scandinavian 50-year-old, attractive, slim, with her breasts jiggling at me. There was a peculiarity to it that made me feel this was a bit strange because I was left with that jiggling image somewhat, but it wasn't erotic. You do get peculiar moments and our access to the patient's body is such a privilege, which is what is also extraordinary about the job.

Yes, I was thinking about the privilege of bathing my baby grand-daughter and how some people never experience that privileged access to a small naked body on their lap.

Yes, extraordinary, and as a doctor you do a lot of it without thinking. You are brought up short when a patient apologizes to you for you having to do a rectal examination, 'I'm so sorry this cannot be what you feel like doing first thing on a Monday morning.' It is the kind of statement you will get and the typical brush off response you will give is, 'It's all in a day's work.'

Now that I'm studying Psychosexual Medicine, I am more aware that sometimes one needs to interpret that embarrassment; it depends on the context of course. That is more difficult and more along the lines of your work, but the advanced training will require it of me. It is learning to use the genital examination as a sort of psychotherapeutic tool. It is interesting that it is usually when you are doing your examination that you may even provoke the emotions that are associated with the presenting condition or problem. It is more difficult to do that with men, but in Psychosexual Medicine you will not just be asking the patient to part their legs so you can conduct your examination, but you will also be observing how that request impacts on them emotionally. This also gives one an advantage over other psychosexual clinicians who are not doctors and therefore cannot have direct physical access to the body. It is very interesting. I am drawn to Psychosexual Medicine because I am interested in what cannot be medically explained and usually there is a mystery to it. There is very poor provision and there are clearly masses and masses of psychosexual problems out there without anywhere near enough treatment resources.

There is a great and huge need. It was at one time my own need, and I went through a bit of that myself when I was having a painful sexual penetrative experience. I did in fact, after several years of confusions, see my own GP and a random gynaecologist at the London Hospital who were both deeply dismissive and unhelpful. In my case it took me until I was 30 to get specialist help, so now whenever I see a 21-year-old I think, 'Hallelujah! You have come early.' Yes, I do think on the whole doctors find it very difficult to talk about sex and I am fairly relaxed now with the healthy fluidity of sexuality, which is important in Psychosexual Medicine. I also know through my own experience and some of my friends as well as my patients that struggling with your sexuality can have a huge impact on your general well-being. Today, there is so much written about how difficult it is to struggle silently with your sexuality and I have personally known more than one lesbian who has killed herself. When I was talking earlier on about my experiences with Luke, the reason I couldn't find anything in the literature about vulval pain was because so little had been written about it then; perhaps one sentence here and there in Gynaecology but too often it is passed over with the suggestion that the woman is very slightly mad. Hence, I have been on a bit of a crusade. It is still a slow process and there are many poorly run psychosexual clinics, the St George's Hospital one is non-existent, to be honest.

Do you find yourself being aware when patients come into the room of whether you find them 'attractive'? I find that when I have a natural attraction to a client, an involuntary chemistry, it becomes easier to move more quickly towards a vibrant discussion, or intimate interaction with them.

Yes, sometimes you think, 'He's quite dishy'. Yes, I say 'he' because I think I am more admiring of women's beauty. I think it is really unusual for an exceptionally attractive man to walk in.

My daughter, whose consulting room is next door will often say, 'Oh, Mum I've just seen someone who is exactly your type, I was tempted to show them straight into your room.'

Yes, I do have a special type, I definitely think my husband is my type physically; I have picked my type of man. Let's say an attractive patient does pitch up and I think 'dishy', but once we are talking about the 'mole', or whatever, I am only into the story of the mole. As a doctor I see the variety, the vagaries of the human body and there is something very normalizing about that. I am sure that it might also temper my own dissatisfactions with my own body, those vagaries compensate for all the media manipulations of the perfect image of the body. I inevitably have opinions about someone's slimness, or their beauty but actually

I am too focused on the diagnosis and on what I am going to find, and that motivation takes over. I have so little time with a patient when I am trying in 10 minutes to gather so much information. It's almost impossible. At the same time I have to stop and regularly take stock that my own experiences are not colouring my judgement of people who present as patients having superficially similar problems. I always have to be careful not to be drawn into misjudgements, or shortcuts that are based on my own vivid experiences.

The time thing is a huge and frustrating factor for NHS doctors in the 21st century.

Yes, it is and it turns the art and science of medicine into an impossible task and the prospects of a Partnership become unappealing. All doctors would say it was an impossible task and I have to accept that I will have to run late because there is no other way. The prospect of doing less is even more unattractive. You are always balancing the justice with the injustices of the whole system but there is just far too much to do and particularly because we have to spend so much more time now ticking boxes, which does not suit me at all. As you will have now discovered I am a little bit complicated and ticking boxes on computers and being bored by the vagaries of NHS bureaucracy does not suit my nature.

8
A COMPREHENSIVE EDUCATION

Vincent studied at the London Hospital (now the Royal London) and is Joint Medical Director of an NHS practice in Brentford.

Were you born in England?

Yes, I was born in 1973, about four miles from where I am now working.

And your parents?

My mum was born in St Vincent in the West Indies and she came to the UK when she was about 16. My father was born in Guyana in South America. They both came over independently and met in London where my mother was doing a nurse training and my father was doing engineering. They married in 1968. Mum started off as a psychiatric nurse and then went on to do a general nurse training at a hospital in Romford. Later, they bought a property in Brentford, where I was brought up with my two brothers. I am the middle one and we were all born close together as my oldest brother is only 10 months older and my youngest one is 15 months younger than me.

Goodness, and your mum had no relatives here to help her?

No. Nobody at all. It must have been extremely tough for her and we have all turned out quite differently and I am the only one to have a vocation and to have followed a profession.

Were you all educated at the same school?

Yes, it was a state Catholic boys' comprehensive. I think as schools go it was a good enough school but academically it wasn't the best in the area, but neither was it the worst. My reflections on looking back, and I was never happy at school, are that it was one of those schools where, if you were really good at sports, you could get away with anything. Unfortunately, I was not brilliant at sports but academically I was in the top five of every year and my focus was always to do well and to become a doctor.

What about your brothers?

My older brother went into recruitment management but he didn't thrive there and now he works for the Metropolitan Police Force. My little brother is someone who has always drifted without any specific focus on life, which strangely has continued into adulthood. He works on the trains as a ticket inspector. I was the only one who had a passion, a vocation from childhood.

Was that related to your mother's nursing career?

I am not sure about that because I have wanted to be a doctor forever and although I may have been influenced by Mum it was actually our family GP more than anything else. There was a big scare, when I was about three, about the whooping-cough vaccine and my parents decided not to inoculate my younger brother who then got whooping-cough as a baby and developed complications, with a serious and brittle asthma. He was back and forth to hospitals throughout our childhood and to our GP's surgery as well. Because we were all three of us still pre-school, it happened that every time Mum took Chris to the GP she had to take us as well. Now I think back about it, I must have spent a lot of time in the GP's surgery as a healthy and curious child. One thing I do remember was that my curious nature was intrigued by everything going on around me. Every time we went to the GP, she would listen to my brother's chest and I would ask Mum what the doctor was listening to. Our GP was fantastic, in fact she only retired recently. In answer to my question she invited me to listen and put her stethoscope to my ears and placed its bell on my chest. Suddenly I could hear my heart beating. It was magic. It must have been around that time I told Mum that I was going to be a doctor when I grew up.

At senior school I loved Classics and ended up doing ancient Greek and Latin but I was also very good at the Sciences and so it just followed on in my mind that I would do Medicine. I was always hard working.

Was your dad proud of you?

I don't know. I suppose the answer is 'yes', but he was never someone that would particularly have shown that emotion at the time. The one thing that happened as I was growing up was the tension between doing well academically and my passion for music, because I was really into music. Somewhere along the line my dad became worried that if I became too good at music I would change my mind and want a music career, which he wouldn't have regarded as a decent and secure career like medicine. To begin with my parents were very supportive when I said I wanted to learn the clarinet and Mum took me to all my lessons. But, after that, when I decided I was going to learn other instruments like the flute they weren't so happy. Mum always went along with everything Dad said so later on I had to save up to buy my own flute and later still my bassoon. The year that I did my GCSEs my dad insisted that I had to give up all my extra-curricular music activities. I was quite good by then and had taken Grade 8 in both instruments and even used to perform the odd clarinet concerto. I was doing loads of concerts and I still do. After some time I realized that, however good I was, there were always zillions of other brilliant clarinet players and flautists but not so with the bassoon. That's why I took it up as my principal instrument and that way I got into loads of orchestras. It has been that way for about 25 years now and it has given me a lot of opportunities as a doctor. I belong to both the European Doctors' Orchestra and to the World Doctors' Orchestra. After I became a houseman with masses of debt the first thing I did was to go out and buy a cello. Yes, I had always wanted a cello but it has only been in the last few years that I have found the time to learn it. I am hoping to take Grade 8 before too much longer.

To go back a bit, as I said, my dad insisted and I stopped doing music the year of my GCSEs but it was a very bad decision for me and I actually found it was harder to study after I had been forced to drop all my music activities. Now I know that I need music to balance my life and that, if I don't have that balance, then it is difficult for me to do the regular study. I made a decision then that I would never give up my music again which, when it came to my A-levels, led to quite a few arguments with Dad. I have always been the one in my family to stand up to my dad. Mum never argued with Dad because what he said went. That was the West Indian way of bringing children up, but I always challenged my father. I cannot tolerate any injustice, and over the years he has mellowed and he is no longer the ogre he once was when we were teenagers. It was Mum who was responsible for raising us. She was only two when her mother died so she was always adamant that when she had her own children she would be there for them in every way, which she was. She taught me to read and write before I went to school and I loved reading with her as a child. Mum had a natural yearning to look after and to help people and I have inherited that from her.

Was there any teacher at school who mentored you in your determination to become a doctor?

No, most of my schooling back then wasn't easy. We were the only black kids in the town and at the school too. Most teachers thought that black kids didn't have the aptitude to be academic. At junior school all the kids were offered the opportunity to learn the violin as part of the curriculum. Later on my parents told me that my oldest brother wanted to do music and to have a violin but the teachers told my parents that black people had no aptitude for music. When it became clear that I was very musical, my parents weren't going to be humiliated again and they found me private tuition. We all played the recorder at primary school and even then it was obvious to those teachers that I was much better than anybody else. Mum brought me my first clarinet. Looking back now I feel a lot of resentment to my teachers but I was strong-willed and it made me more determined to prove myself and to become a doctor. I was often unhappy during my schooling with the endless tensions between the sports brigade time wasters, who never wanted to study, and academia and the fact that nobody there was interested in guiding me. I had so much difficulty choosing my subjects on my own and although I went for three Sciences, if I had my time over again with what I now know, I would have chosen Chemistry, Latin and Greek. My A-levels were two years of undiluted misery.

Did you just think 'doctor' or did you have an idea of what kind of doctor you wanted to be?

I just thought 'doctor' until I started at medical school and then I thought I would become an obstetrician.

Oh! Well, first tell me where you trained?

I trained at the London Hospital, as it was then called in the East End. I did go up to look at the Cambridge colleges, where I sat on the lawn with three other people from public school and feeling very out of place. I think it was my mum who must have talked to me about specialties and I remember her saying, 'Obstetrics is quite good because everyone is always having babies.' As soon as I did my obstetric rota I changed my mind. It was a horrible time for me because I just kept worrying about all the things that could go wrong and I had seen quite a few disasters. I just thought, 'This is awful - you go into hospital to have a baby you just assume you will come out with a healthy baby – but when that baby dies and you are the doctor at the other end of the line, that is too awful.' Then, I had a crisis of confidence and just had no idea of what I was going to end up doing.

A COMPREHENSIVE EDUCATION

Were you the only black student?

Oh no, there were two others, not counting all the Asians, but they both came from really wealthy families and stuff. I didn't have much to do with them. By the time I got to medical school it was not acceptable to express overt racism but people still had no hesitation in expressing elitism or sexism. The overwhelming thing I felt was that I was out of place because I had gone to a comprehensive and not to a public school. One of the first people I talked to was a girl who thought that, because I hadn't gone to public school I had no right to be at medical school, and her opinion was shared by a lot of the students – this was 1991.

I found it hard, as it was all bookwork for the first two years and it was hard. Medicine is hard work and unlike today's students, we didn't then do proper clinical stuff until the third year. I think that was quite good because it gives you time to grow up just that little bit, which makes the difference before you properly have patient contact. Also, you get rid of the people who don't want to be there. Unfortunately, we had a suicide in my first year of someone who always wanted to be a fireman but his parents wouldn't let him. I found that very disturbing.

I did have to work hard to get through the pre-clinical, but by the time we were on the wards it all changed for me when I found that I had a natural gift for clinical medicine. Suddenly, I was so much better than most of the other students. What's interesting is that the people I am still close to now - my close friends - not one of them went to public school. It's funny how we found ourselves, we filtered down into a group and we have all had good careers. Three of them are consultants now and three of us are senior GPs and I am also a GP trainer and have registrars training with me at the practice. The guy who is my best friend actually went to Cambridge from a comprehensive and he had a miserable time there. We've only talked briefly about his experience but I look at him and think, 'That could have been me.' He only started to enjoy himself when he got to the London Hospital.

How do you understand your ability to have above average communication skills?

I've always been curious and good at relating to people since I was a kid and there was a big thing at the London about teaching communications skills. When I became a GP trainer, and later on when I became a tutor in communication skills, my take on it was that it is something that is very difficult to teach if you don't have a natural and warm curiosity about people. My mum always put other people before herself right up until the moment she died. It was this time last year that she became so ill and she died at the beginning of September. I am still not sure if that can be taught. There are a lot of people who think if you are good at the sciences you should go into medicine but I don't agree. I think medicine is a vocation and if you have that in you then you will get through medical school regardless of all the rote studying you have to do. I think I got that passion to care for people from my mother but she has passed away now. My father has never been like that. That yearning, that feeling of wanting to help people has always been inside of me. Yes, learning how to deal with live patients was what interested me most during my training.

When we were first on the wards and learning how to take histories we had to work in pairs. I remember one of the first patients that I had to interview with my partner Kate. We were talking to this woman and we were taking her social history when she started crying. We just didn't know what to do to make her better but we got out the tissues. The reason she was crying was because she had lost her son in an industrial accident years and years ago but she had never spoken about it before. It was pretty horrific because we felt we didn't have the skills to help her. Now that I am a GP it happens a lot. I always remember how I felt out of my depth the first time I met that avalanche of human emotion and how helpless I felt. I am recalling another occasion when I first qualified and wanted everyone to know that I was a doctor. I was at an airport and they called out over the public-address system, 'Is there a doctor in the vicinity?' I rushed over to the information desk where I found a very sick child but to my embarrassment, it was ages since I had done Paediatrics, and I really didn't know what to do.

The feeling that you want to make somebody better but you cannot, is it hard to learn as a young doctor?

Yes, it is hard. One of the hardest experiences I had as a medical student was when I was doing Paediatrics and the firm that I was attached to was at the Queen Elizabeth Children's Hospital in Hackney on the Gastro-Oncology ward. Knowing that almost none of those children would grow up to be adults, well it was horrible because every single child had some awful diagnosis. I found it the most heartbreaking thing that I have ever had to do. It upset me so much when I went home to think of a beautiful child who was never going to grow up.

I imagine that might also have been the emotion when you realized that your mother was terminally ill. Were you able to look after her when she died, I don't mean to be her doctor?

Well, I was her doctor too, pretty much. It was this time last year. She had had breast cancer years ago – yes it was just after I qualified in '97 – when I was working in Chelmsford on a breast firm. She was then clear for years and years until she developed another primary tumour about two years ago but she didn't recover as was expected. When they investigated further, after a difficult and unresponsive chemo treatment, she was found to have another inoperable primary tumour on her pancreas. The reason I took on my job in Essex was to be nearer to her as I was working in Hackney and Harley Street at the time. I remember coming back to the surgery in Hackney for an afternoon session after taking her and Dad – my parents don't drive – for her diagnosis and being quite upset. I had been dumped on by the senior partner and found I had twice as many patients and I may have been a bit short with the receptionist. A few days later the senior partner pulled me up: 'I've had a complaint from the receptionist that you didn't say "Hello" when you came in to work.' I told him that I was sorry and explained about my mother and her terminal diagnosis but his response was to reprimand me: 'Whatever was going on in your personal life, we don't want you bringing it to work, and you must remember that stress doesn't exist in doctors during professional hours.' 'You bastard' is actually what I thought. 'You are a doctor and you are telling me this, you have no empathy.' I decided to look around for another job, which I did and that is where I now work. The sad thing about leaving Hackney was leaving the patients because, as a good doctor in a bad practice, you are still able to look after your patients well, but my mother was my world. I felt she had invested so much in me growing up, not so much my dad, but if anything ever happened to my mum I was going to be there for her. At my current practice they kept offering me time off but it wasn't needed until Mum got really ill at the end of August and she ended up having a syringe driver.

Nevertheless, one of the memories that will go with me all my life happened at the Hackney practice, where continuity of care was always very important to me. I have never been interested in the 10-minute session, which comes to an end when the door closes and you may never see that patient again. I remember one of the days when I was feeling especially low about Mum and this couple came in to see me with their autistic young son. He was about 10. I am sure that I did not reveal that I was at low ebb that afternoon, and my young patient had not spoken a single word to anyone. At the end of the session he came right over and gave me a huge hug.

That is so moving. Sorry, to go back to the earlier thoughts, what is a syringe driver? I have noticed how serious illness often introduces unfamiliar and unwelcome words into our vocabularies.

Mum was vomiting a great deal and the hospice staff came to see her at home and decided that she had to have a continuous pump where the drugs are maintained subcutaneously. My dad was beside himself when he saw the driver apparatus being put up. I knew I needed to be there on that Friday night and then Mum asked me to stay. My intention was to go back to London the next day but Mum just gave me this look, which said, 'I don't want you to go.' Mum had never asked anything of me before, and from that day I didn't leave the house until she died two weeks later. We had the hospice team coming, the district nurse, and relatives, left, right and centre. It was very traumatic and I knew that I was needed. I looked after the house, did all the cooking and cleaning, liaised with everyone. Yes, it was stressful. Dad turned 70 last year and has his own health problems. Overnight we would have a Macmillan 'sitter' who came every night and when she left at 5.30 am I would take over until my older brother Jason arrived, having got his family off to school. I was by Mum's side when she died and I feel very privileged to have done that.

Obviously, she was there when I came into the world, and I was there when she left. I think Mum always loved us just the same but each of us always felt jealous that she loved one of us more than the other.

Ultimately, I think I was the one she was the most proud of and the one she felt most secure with. I was always the one to sort everything out in our family.

What time of day did she die?

It was just after six on a Sunday night and it was very interesting because we had had a nurse with us all day and then, when she left, Mum just passed peacefully away. I had wept all my tears before she died and I just went into organizational mode. The most upsetting thing for me was when our parish priest came to give her the Last Rites. That was a difficult time for me.

Her death must still seem very new.

Yes, just a year ago and I don't spend a lot of time thinking about her now because it still upsets me. Your mother – well, if you are lucky – your mother is the person who nurtures you all your life. It's interesting because, although I was really close to Mum, I was probably also the most independent of all her children and I was always the one who wanted to get out of the house and make my own way in life. I guess we shared that medical thing together, which Mum always understood, as she had worked in the medical profession all of her life, albeit as a nurse. I have always been very independent and in fact I found it very difficult going home for the university holidays. Yes, it was difficult because they reacted badly if I was out past midnight – they had no idea what I got up to at medical school – but they replied, 'Yes, yes, but you are here now.'

How sad for you to think that she had grown up motherless.

Exactly. I didn't cry when she died, although I cried a lot at the funeral. What was really helpful was the fact that work was so supportive. They gave me the time off to be with her, unlike the job in Hackney where I would probably have got the sack for taking those weeks off.

How did you feel about your mother's treatment and did she have to have more chemotherapy?

Yes, they treated her with chemo for the second round of breast cancer and it made her very sick and ill. When they discovered the pancreatic tumour they offered Mum more chemo. I saw that look of dread in her eyes because she just didn't have the strength any more, but she still agreed to it because Dad wanted her to have it. I remember the oncologist tried to sell it to Mum by saying that, unlike with the breast cancer, this time it would be more targeted. I remember her last chemo appointment when I sat with her on the oncology unit for that last hour-and-a-half of Mum submitting. Dad was really upbeat but I saw that look in Mum's eyes and knew she was desperate not to have any more chemo. I remember that she had a new oncologist and he looked through her notes and said, 'I don't think this is helping you.' My dad was very upset but he hadn't faced up to the fact that she had an inoperable cancer, whereas as soon as I heard that she had pancreatic cancer I knew that was it. I think that is one of the worst things about being a doctor hearing that someone you love has been given a terminal diagnosis. You know that it's curtains. Yes, that is that! Mum, being medical, also knew the truth.

She confided all her last wishes to me, and how she wanted her funeral to be conducted, but Dad was in denial. This is where I got really angry about the whole communications aspect and how nobody had communicated properly to my dad. As I said, he was an engineer and he wanted to believe that doctors were there to fix things. My dad is an intelligent man and if somebody had sat him down and explained to him, stage by stage, what was going to happen but nobody did that for him. Too often as a profession we wrap things up in cotton wool and things that need to be said are not said, which made it harder for Dad to accept that she was dying. He never had a proper conversation with her, and when that end-of-life syringe driver went up, I wanted him to speak to her before it was too late.

It feels very privileged that you have shared this experience about your mother's illness and death with me and I am imagining that what you have been sharing with me now informs how you deal with such difficult moments professionally.

That is true, and funnily enough I held that opinion even before this happened with Mum, so it hasn't so much as changed the way I work as much as reinforced it. I do wonder if perhaps the doctors thought that I was able to translate the situation to my parents but that makes me feel quite angry. Mum knew what the deal was and I knew but my dad didn't, which just reinforced my belief that bad news is bad news. A lot of people forget that. If you don't actually and physically put into words the fact that someone is going to die, then the partner or children may feel cheated. In terminal diagnoses you are not just dealing with the patient but their family as well and after Mum's death Dad became very resentful. One of the reasons that I think I am a good GP, and I don't think I am blowing my own trumpet here, is because despite being taught various models of consultation skills I always regard my patients as individuals. When I am training my registrars I want them to understand that if they are speaking to two patients but using an identical communication model, then there is something wrong. No two people are alike and you have to find the right way of approaching each of your patients individually and learn to adapt your consultation style to fit every context.

Something I've noticed while we have been talking is that you refer to yourself as crying. You use the verb 'I cried'. In my conclusion, which I wrote before I was given this welcome opportunity to interview you, I talk about how hard it is for men to cry...

The funny thing is that I am not a weepy person and I only ever cried as a small boy but there are some moments where you are just taken back to being that small child who has hurt their knee and then the only way you can express the current emotion is by crying. Yes, I remember when Mum was effectively lying on her deathbed and unbeknown to me Dad had gone up to the cathedral to find a priest to administer the Last Rites. He went round to the Bishop's secretary's office and one of the nuns – I went to a Catholic school – who taught me, went to call Father Grant.

Father Grant used to be the parish priest when I was still involved in the church, singing in the choir and serving at the altar and all that sort of stuff. The doorbell went and I left Mum's bedside to open the door and there was Father Grant and Sister Eleanor, who taught me when I was seven or eight. As soon as

DOCTORS DISSECTED

I saw Sister Eleanor standing there I knew why they had come and I became that seven-year-old boy again. I started crying and I couldn't stop. I wouldn't normally do that and it certainly wouldn't ever happen to me at work but it was just something involuntary that happened. My dad didn't shed a tear and neither did my brothers. I knew I would be fine but my father and brothers didn't know what to say to me. The thing is that when you start crying there is the awful fear that you will never stop, but the tears have to come.

Yes, that is exactly what some of my clients say to me, they are afraid to cry because they might never stop. I have just remembered that another of the contributors in the book talks about how her mother's only dying request was to have Mozart's Clarinet Concerto played at her funeral. I wonder what you, as a musician, feel when you hear it as music is something that can even put those men who find it hard to express emotion in touch with their feelings?

Well, yes, that was one of the things that I immediately thought of after she died, although Mum didn't ask for anything other than specific hymns, but she did ask to be cremated. For me there was no option other than to chose the second movement of the Mozart Clarinet Concerto to accompany her coffin to the chute, as it was something that I had played to her several times as a teenager. There was no question of it, and that is what Mum had at the very end. She loved to hear me play it, and had it not have been her funeral I would have played it myself.

9
THERE IS A CANDLE IN YOUR HEART

After being dismissed from the NHS for 'whistleblowing', Zoe now works in private practice. She was born in 1941.

I have often wondered why I became a doctor because it was a totally weird choice coming from my background. My father was chairman of British American Tobacco Company and my mother had been brought up on Park Avenue by a man who had made American history when his product had the single largest launch of any product hitherto made in the States, and it was the book-match.

The book-match?

Yes, the book-match – matches! I have never smoked, which shows you I have never felt part of the family. I was born in Saigon, at the beginning of the war, and in fact left on the last boat which was not torpedoed by the Japanese. All subsequent boats were lost. My mother was due to give birth to me and they would not let her on to the ship so she drank a bottle of gin and got somebody with a jeep to drive her over an uneven road until it stimulated labour. I was born drunk as Mother ran with an unwashed baby to the boat as it was about to pull out of harbour. I was sent from Cairo, where we were living, to boarding school in England and thereafter I only saw my parents for holidays. They became strangers.

DOCTORS DISSECTED

I was a challenging child who was continually being thrown out of the convents for being uncontrollable. My mother appealed to me to finish my education without being expelled one more time as she had become bored of sewing on nametapes. I started to learn to pretend, to pretend to conform. My academic report was superlative but there was also a line that said, 'Zoe has a tendency to exhibitionism, which she will control only when she wants to.' At the beginning of sixth form there was an announcement, 'Would those girls doing Sciences go the right and the Arts pupils to the left.' Although I had an arts type brain there was no way I was going to follow my school nemesis, Brenda Tandy into Arts, so I joined the Science Sixth. I got stuck with sciences, which I was good at but they were unbelievably boring. One day a girl visited the convent and everybody thought she was wonderful because she was a doctor and I wanted to be wonderful too, instead of being known as the difficult child, and that was that.

There was no sense of vocation?

None whatsoever. I had no idea what I was taking on. Now, I love being a doctor, I still adore it. I loved the elegance of learning how to make a diagnosis. I trained at St Thomas's Hospital in 1960 and I was soon drawn to Psychiatry, but I discovered that it was very formulaic, full of meaningless words, so I decided to go into Neurology once I qualified. I continue to be fascinated by the interface between the mind and the brain.

I was taught brilliantly. I was lucky, I was among the last bunch of medical students who had brilliant teaching and particularly in Neurology but everything has since changed. Medical students are no longer taught how to examine a patient and how to take a proper history. Now, they just do all the tests without a preliminary and thorough examination and the NHS is wasting so much money. We were taught to use our eyes and senses and to observe the patient but they do not train students to make a diagnosis any more, or how to interpret results and so they chuck unnecessary and crazily expensive tests around like confetti.

It sounds as if you became a different sort of student at medical school.

I really loved the romance of saving lives but I still had the lure of going into Neurology and wanting to learn more about the brain and in Neurology you do not 'save lives', because so often there is no cure. As my career progressed it got interspersed with marriages but in terms of the patient/doctor relationship I became more interested in the individual, in the setting of their illness, rather than wanting to be the clever doctor. I stayed on at Thomas's and did my house jobs there, and after I qualified I went on a circuit of London teaching-hospitals and went on to become a Senior Neurology Registrar.

At that point, in 1980 there were 28 'time expired'* neurology registrars who were waiting for promotion and no consultant jobs available because the whole politics of medicine changed and money had gone to the local health authorities who said, 'Goody, goody, we can do without neurologists because they do nothing. Neurology can be fitted into general medicine.' This was before you could treat multiple sclerosis and that is why MS is such a mess in this country because general physicians are not qualified to make the diagnosis. At that point I had married a man whose wife had died with three children, so I decided my life would be better suited to working in NHS general practice.

---

* Registrars who have completed their two-year training contract but have not found a consultant vacancy and who end up in limbo.

DOCTORS DISSECTED

Do you have children?

No, I only have stepchildren and anyway my husband left me and I looked after his children. I was left with three kids. It was crazy and I was stony broke. I used to do night emergencies as well to cover the costs. After they grew up, I married a surgeon whom I had known as a medical student and who had children and he didn't want any more children either, so it never happened. That marriage lasted about five years and during it I came back into hospital medicine. Unfortunately, it was an abusive marriage and I think my husband – who was a brilliant but self made man, a surgeon who challenged the boundaries and made science headlines – was also determined to marry an up-market lady and that was me. At the same time I threatened his anxieties about class and for being who I was and he became abusive. There were little things I had to learn like I could never go through a door first because if I went through a door first and he followed he would hear everyone greeting me and not him, and then he would beat me up later that night. I always had to come second. It was so, so sad because he was also a great guy, a brilliant surgeon and I was very fond of him.

He demanded that I was always properly dressed which meant being expensively dressed and I was even forced to wear a mink coat, and I don't like mink at all. I couldn't even read a book if he hadn't heard about it, he tore up a novel by Iris Murdoch because he had never heard her name. He was a complete control freak and he ended up dying of Parkinson's disease.

What did it feel like working as a neurologist by day and being infantilized every night?

It was difficult, very difficult. Professional marriages can become like a prison – you don't dare to tell anyone because it is like a

204

betrayal. The abuse crept up, it didn't happen all at once, the abuse was gradual but it was frightening.

How old were you by then? It is hard to get any sense of timing as I listen.

I was in my late thirties, so I had already done a lot of medicine and come back from general practice to hospital medicine.

Do you now make any links between your husband's personality disorder and his ending up with a neurological disease?

No, I think it was his personality, and eventually he got an agitated depression and he started drinking very heavily. He was also mainlining with Valium but he didn't seem to make any surgical mistakes in theatre. He was still president of this and president of that but he became physically violent with me. I knew that I was turning him into a monster who had to dominate me and I knew it was time to end our marriage of attraction and hatred.

What sort of effect did this second marital failure have on you? If I am following correctly you were not even 40 by then.

I just knew that I wasn't going to try again, and that I was too bruised. I think also, looking back now, the story of my romantic life is that I have never got over my first ever boyfriend, J; although I have tried my best he still occupies my mind. He was at Thomas's with me and we were the dazzling student couple of our time. I was a Catholic virgin when I met him and I thought if somebody slept with you they married you, but he didn't. I was a virgin until I was 20 and it was an amazing relationship in every way until he took me to a pub after we had been together for three years and told me that he was in fact engaged to be married to a girl he had left behind in Australia and so we would have to end our relationship. I became icy cold and I remember thinking, 'Why aren't the walls of this pub falling in?' I am now remembering that sensation of panic. Terrible. I was a houseman at 'Tommies' so we still had to see each other every day. I became a walking zombie and one of his friends told me that I looked as if I was going to die of grief and he invited me out for a drink. He proceeded to tell me that J had shared his experience of taking my virginity with every member of the rowing team. I thought to myself, and I still don't know if this was salacious gossip or true, 'You have taken my innocence. Now I shall walk on the dark side.' I became wildly promiscuous and would only sleep with men who wanted sex; I wanted nothing to do with love. I was a small fish in a very big pond and I became wild, wild, wild. It was a scream, a terrible scream, of pain.

It seems there has always been and there still is a strong sense of individuality and even anarchy at the centre of your personality and a natural tendency as the headmistress observed to act out your feelings.

Yes, I was still at heart a boarding school child and not given to reflection in my private life. I am still no good at complaining, no good at all, I just put all the pain and disappointment somewhere else. It is interesting how psychic splitting occurs and how doctors are often very good examples of living two kinds of emotional lives. Nevertheless, I have continued to love J all my life and he also became one of the most successful surgeons in the country. St Thomas's has produced some great surgeons. It has not been at all easy and our lives have continued in a seesaw of intimacy and absence over the last 40 years but with far, far more absences during which time he has gone on to have a very successful marriage. He was my first ever boyfriend and I am still imprinted with him, psychologically, physically, entirely and after the last dumping I became a Buddhist. I am fascinated by religion – not by the performance of religion – but the mysticism of religion, I love it.

Goodness it is such intense stuff and I need to catch up and think. Was it that being a boarding school girl with very poor childhood parental attachments and disappointments in love that turning to religion, to mysticism was…

I think the parallel of religion had always been there. As a child in the convent I would look into the flame of the candle and see eternity. I learnt the Gospels by heart as a child because I was so bored, I was bored out of my head at school even in the sixth form. So, I had no problems learning the long and complex chants and prayers in Buddhism, which are sublime. There is a sort of mysticism that has always been a parallel mother to me if you like which has held me close and stopped me becoming insane.

I was at a preparatory convent school and even there, there were a couple of nuns who 'held' me and who have never left me or my inner world and then there was the priest. Oh, God, I must have been six or seven and I thought that this priest was already dead and had come from Heaven to teach us. He had a skinny little neck and a big white collar and white, white hair and watery-blue eyes and his name was Father Damian. When he came in we all stood up and he made us put our hands on the desk and put our heads down as he said, 'Now remember God is in Heaven and he is all around you and he is within you and he loves you and that is all that matters.' Ah! I loved him and so I had my imaginary friend who was called God but he might have been called Dog. It would not have mattered because I knew that he loved me and I could talk to him through the medium of the candle and that has always sustained me, that flame of meditation. The universe has always fascinated me; it has never left me and it is the unity of my life.

Were you observant during medical school?

I went to church…but as soon as sex hits you which was quite late, I used to go to church regularly but then I decided that sex was much more interesting. Not just sex but the thought of a real person caring for you instead of my imaginary person. I didn't then know that I was only destined to meet bastards. I still have nightmares about my relationship with J and they always repeat the same story. J is doing a ward round with his students and I try to catch his eye but he ignores me, or laughs at me and walks away. I wake up in a sweat and it still happens to me about every two months as it has done for 15 years.

You have loved this man for more than 50 years?

Yes, it is a love story and I have talked to different therapists ad nauseam about it for years.

Can we go back to the way you have found consolation in religion?

Yes, I converted.

THERE IS A CANDLE IN YOUR HEART

Was it a reaction to your broken heart?

No, it was as a regression, as a result of failing to have mature human relationships. I was emotionally illiterate.

Do you still regard yourself as emotionally illiterate?

In relation to myself yes, but no, not for others. I will not advise my patients on their marriages and I tell everyone that I have had two divorces and I am no use at that. I believe that people should be married but I am not skilled at helping them to get that particular conversation going. I try to keep people in marriages unless they are simply awful. I tried to compromise but I still failed.

You mentioned before we started recording that you have had cancer. You say that you were a boarding school girl who didn't talk about feelings but perhaps your body has reacted to these powerful betrayals. I am sure you know Henry Maudsley's wise adage: 'The sorrow which has no vent in tears may make other organs weep.'

Yes, but you have to remember that I was also on hormones all my life: I took the pill and then I took hormone replacement therapy (HRT) so I belong to the generation that over-oestrogenized itself. What the medical profession did to women was terrible: anybody who is anybody would have had the clue if they had done the simplest bit of research on populations and the distribution of breast cancer. Since the millennia breast cancer is what happens to the rich and to the fat and it does not happen to the skinny unless it is a triple negative type of cancer. Breast cancer is also the disease of contamination and pollution. We didn't know about oestrogen receptors in the old days but now that we do it is on the door, obvious to everyone except the pharmaceuticals, that you do not put a female on to hormones for the whole of her life and expect her not to have cancer. Even now it is quite amazing that the epidemic is not even greater. I remember when I was going down to theatre for the mastectomy thanking my breast for the lovely experiences it had given me. I had a dialogue with my breast about my lovers. Sex is a language but I don't miss it now, just like I don't miss alcohol.

Why did you take HRT? I was always too suspicious to do so?

Well, as I said, we did not know about oestrogen receptors then and I only took it when my hot flushes were making it impossible for me to work and I thought it made me feel better. But it was all psychological because when I stopped taking it later on it made no difference and the symptoms returned. The only thing that I have since reflected is that my brother is bipolar and I have also been prone to swings of depression, which I think that frankly I have earned the right to; I have got a lot to be depressed about. I must be allowed my grief, but then I started getting grief that was not analyzable and which would come down like a fog, so now I am on antidepressants. Before I came off the oestrogen I never had such deep depression as I suffer now, so I still don't know if the oestrogen also acted as a defence against the bipolar cycle.

Is it correct to say bipolar because it sounds as if when you are not depressed you are okay?

I am fine but I can be high, I can go through two nights working hard and suddenly getting everything done. I have always had an erratic energy. I will have moods in which I am not unhappy but it is a complete dislocation between myself and anything and everything. I feel as if a fog has come between everything and me. If I go to a dinner party I will smile through my teeth and make a huge effort, but I have to fall back on acting, I am very skilled at acting, but then I will leave and return willingly into the welcoming dark. I love that bit of T. S. Eliot where he says: 'O dark dark dark. They all go into the dark.' I live by the *Four Quartets*. Sometimes, when I am mad and suicidal I talk to this great oak tree in Windsor Park, which has been present since the time of Henry VIII. I look at it and I think this tree is covered in fairies and it has such strength. It is old and has just got a trunk left now with a few bits coming off it but I feel the strength coming out and that is my reference point.

I trained as an actress and that was also primarily to escape the trauma of my childhood but I have found that the wounds can never go, only be partially healed.

Yes, that is what I also learnt from my psychoanalyses – if you are a mouse be a good mouse and do not try to be an elephant. Live your own truth. Embrace life. I learnt not to be ashamed of my childhood and I have forgiven my parents because they did not know what they were doing. My mother desperately wanted a beautiful daughter whom she could dress up. She always wore couture and even when she was older she could wear rags and look amazing, she was incredibly beautiful. I am not and never have been interested in any of that. I was a disappointment to my mother, and she wasn't interested in me being academically successful.

DOCTORS DISSECTED

Did your parents have any interest in your professional life?

None at all.

None?

No, nothing. When Dad was dying, both of them died under my watch, I was looking after him. It was quite sweet because gradually other patients on the ward saw our names were the same and put two and two together. They would go up to his bed and say, 'Do you know, she's good. A very good doctor.' Both my parents were alcoholics and Dad was on the Liver ward that Hammersmith Hospital then shared with the Neurology ward. He finally got some good reports of me. My mother was a gutsy lady. I always thought of her as Tallulah Bankhead – you couldn't stand up against her – it was quite impossible.

When did you return to a spiritual life?

After my divorce I went back to church and was trying to take it seriously in spite of the paedophile problems and so on. I went back to my alma mater, which was Farm Street, but I was already intellectually involved in all the writings of the Buddha, Sufis and other important philosophers.

I was looking after the Queen Mother of Oman with a group of physicians. I came to love her to pieces and she selected me to be her physician. I would see her every month both in Oman and London where I looked after her for about five years until 1982. Then, one day I was looking after her in Salalah and she went into heart failure. One of the problems of being royal is that when you get really sick your local doctors disappear, as they don't want to be associated with a royal death or failure, so they disappear. I was left looking after her and she was blue and frothing at the mouth but the right medical kit was there and I did all the right things. She asked me to stay with her all that day while so many family members visited her and she gave out counsel. At the end she was white and sweating with fatigue and I said, 'It is all very well, you looking after everyone but who looks after you?' She looked at me with such anger, anger like I had never seen as she sat up on her pillows with such power, it seemed to come suddenly and from nowhere and she replied, 'Allah.' I thought, I don't know what that power is but I want it, I want it for myself.

A spiritual pathway has always been my strength and I now see the Buddhist faith as one that is also death friendly. I already had a heightened sense of the importance of the individual, what the individual becomes, but now I also have a sense of the unimportance of the individual when you look at the immensity of creation, and of how very little we know.

I cannot go through a day without thinking about death, but perhaps not with the equanimity that you do.

I think about death every day and not unhappily. I have been trained how to be a companion to my patient from diagnosis to death and I have often put the bad news explicitly, in that I will say, 'I am afraid I have got bad news for you, this is a malignancy and it is a bad one. We are going to fight this tooth-and-nail all the way and I will not leave you, I will be there for you, whatever.' That is 'my-speak', and I try to make it humorous, or even funny as I did with my best friend who I diagnosed with a terminal sarcoma. When she was dying I made sure that she was cared for by the local oncology team so that I could see her frequently. They found it weird because among dying people there is a certain meditative stillness except when I came into the room and was with her. Then there was high jinx as we celebrated the life that we had lived over the years. The Palliative Care Consultant thought we were completely nuts. My friend said, 'I think I must be getting worse because the doctors have stopped examining me.' That is a classic. I felt her belly and there were these terrible craggy lumps of everything; it was horrible and I said, 'Oh! Veronica, they have made a wrong diagnosis, do you know that you are pregnant?' She was 66. 'But this is not going to be a baby, it is an angel because I can feel the wings.' This was our metaphor for her death. I would come in to see her every day and say, 'Those wings are getting stronger and stronger, and you will soon be able to fly.' I helped her quietly into death. I like trying to do that with everybody. You can die and it can be like giving birth, it can be another kind of living.

I have no fear of death because my candle's flame says there is eternity. And the magnificence of the universe…well the Higgs Boson at Cerne was discovered last year and I was dancing a jig in my consulting room saying, 'The Higgs has been discovered, they have just announced it.' Most of my patients hadn't a clue what I was talking about but it was the most important thing ever – if it was not for the Higgs Boson we would be particles going into wherever…we would not have mass. My patient just looked at me and said, 'You are nuts and I have got this pain that I want you to diagnose.' I love science because I love anything that we discover about the universe, about creation, I am fascinated by it all. I am determined not to get Alzheimer's, so I can learn more.

What we have learnt about the brain is that everything is connected to everything else and, whereas we thought it had fixed pathways, we know better now and that although certain things are fixed there are also many things that are not hard wired, and it is all about these connections. I have a theory about Alzheimer's but it is probably not right because Iris Murdoch died of it but what we call a lot of Alzheimer's is probably just people in silent despair, old people who have given up: they watch the TV, they become couch potatoes, they have been left alone, and ignored rather like neglected children and they implode. How do you accurately diagnose Alzheimer's when you require very skilled and selective scanning to do so? It seems to me that nearly all the people who have been, and are now more and more being warehoused as having the disease probably do not, they are wrongly diagnosed and many old people have just given up hope.

We have also learnt how the parents' loving gaze and their feedback affect the infant brain, the impact of which lasts throughout life.

Everything matters for children because that is how they lay their brains down and you cannot lay a brain down by isolating or ignoring a child because if they are neglected they get poor synapses and they may end up violent. Children need maximum plasticity. It doesn't matter what that is, and nobody could say I was ever violent because although I was unhappy as a child I still had all sorts of experiences. It doesn't matter what just so long as you are making many different connections with the world. Nobody could say my childhood was boring.

And you had your priest?

Yes, I had my priest; I had God. I had completely mad teachers and hobbies and adventures and I also knew even as a child that I had to get out of school and into the world and to live with every breath.

10
MARTIN'S
CONSULTING ROOM

The emphasis in medical ethics on sexual correctness is not so much to restrict the doctor as to offer a promise to the patient: a promise which is far more than a reassurance that he or she will not be taken advantage of. It is a positive promise of physical intimacy without a sexual basis. Yet what can such intimacy mean? Surely it belongs to the experiences of childhood. We submit to the doctor by quoting to ourselves a state of childhood.

John Berger, *A Fortunate Man*

Searching for this quotation in an extraordinary book which is an account of a family GP, John Sassal, working in a remote rural community in the 1960s,* my thoughts glide to a recent hour when I took my adolescent grandson, Dan, to my own GP and friend, whom I knew would find the time to listen. Recent and traumatic events in his life have caused anxiety to stir and even to break through Dan's characteristic adolescent and invincible sense of immortality; perhaps his first existential stirrings of dread about his mortality. I knew that this important psychosomatic consultation would require more time than would be available at his besieged NHS practice in Brighton where even a 10-minute consultation must be regarded as a gift.

We are sitting in my doctor's waiting room. Dan is waiting on two counts: the first is that he will hear, later today, whether or not he has made it to Cambridge; and the second is to discuss his

---

* Tragically and ironically, some years after the book was published Sassal suffered so severely from depression that he shot himself.

gut, whose innocuous sounding symptoms are concerning him rather more than me. He is not used to consulting doctors, or worrying about whether his body is working properly and he assures me that his anticipation of this unusual visit to a doctor is stressing him out far more than his entrance results. I happen to believe him as he also suffers from needle phobia. Flustered, he turns to me, 'I hope he won't ask me to take all my clothes off, will he? Will he touch my stomach? I am not going to have a blood test, am I? I shall refuse.' Then, having observed an emaciated and jaundiced woman emerge from the surgery, Dan has a sudden and raw realization expressed as rapid-fire questions. 'Doctors must spend a lot of their lives having to tell people very unpleasant and difficult things that they don't really want to hear, mustn't they? Don't you think that must affect the doctor almost as much as his patient? Is it something they can ever just get used to doing? How would you begin tell somebody that they were dying?'

I don't trust doctors. It's not to say there ain't some good ones, but on a general level, no, I wouldn't trust 'em at all.
Keith Richards

The best doctors seem to have a sixth sense about disease. They feel its presence, know it to be there, perceive its gravity before any intellectual process can define, catalogue and put it into words. Patients sense this about such a physician as well: that he is attentive, alert, ready, that he cares. No student of medicine should miss observing such an encounter. Of all the moments in medicine this one is most filled with drama, with feeling, with history.
Michael La Combe, *Annals of Internal Medicine* (1993)

DOCTORS DISSECTED

As I welcome a patient into my consulting room, a decade plus after the millennium, I have a flashback to my room in the late 1970s, 35 years ago. Today, the welcome is the same: pleasantries, or a chat to put them at ease and catch up on events since our last consultation of weeks, months, maybe a year ago. There is a problem – maybe a symptom of pain – lower back perhaps, or vaguely abdominal. My core procedures are unchanged: I take a history, which is followed by clinical examination. No shortcuts as I ask for the exact history, when did their symptom start, what does the pain feel like, the distribution, does it come and go, what helps? I like to take a very exact and detailed oral history that will include every aspect, and subtle nuance, which all takes time.

The biggest change the time traveller would see is the arrival of the computer screen and keyboard on my desk. The trolley with the blood tubes and specimen bottles is unchanged, the drawers containing dressings and other supplies are the same as ever. It is all familiar but on the desk there is no longer a patient's file, just a bare sheet of paper for clinical notes, which will be scanned and then shredded. Somehow the hand-written record, when viewed later on a screen, evokes at a stroke the details of an earlier consultation in my mind with maybe a sketch included to describe or encapsulate the clinical examination. That computer terminal embodies the change between when I started to the present time for it has become the portal to all the new technologies, which follow the initial clinical examination.

I had a sobering experience this week of the kind that makes you re-evaluate everything you are doing. I received a delayed report about a patient of mine who had undergone an operation three months ago that resulted in the cure of her symptoms. She had been so chronically unwell that she was unable to work for the past year or two. The worrying aspect for me was that one month before the operation I had told her that her problems were all due to depression, or some form of psychological disorder; she had not liked this at all and had told me so. I have known this woman since she was a child. On one occasion, as a young adult, she suffered from giardiasis; giardia is a single celled parasite that can make people ill with chronic gastroenteritis. This was cured, but when she was in her thirties she frequently complained that she had caught it again, although we were never able to prove this as her symptoms, which tended to come and go, remained unexplained.

Two years ago, she arrived with lower abdominal pain and although the picture was not typical the working diagnosis was appendicitis; after CT scanning proved the diagnosis she underwent an appendectomy. Her progress was far from smooth, and then there were months of night sweats, back pain, exhaustion and weight loss which demanded further investigations, and there followed a series of referrals to a gynaecologist, a gastroenterologist, an infectious diseases expert and various radiologists who carried out scans by ultrasound, MRI and CT but all without a diagnosis being made. During that time my patient started to complain of widespread itching, to the extent that she became obsessed with the thought of having scabies; she was also unable to sleep, was tearful, had panic attacks, and continued to lose weight.

Eventually, after presenting in the emergency room of a central London hospital, she was seen by a gastroenterology specialist who concluded that despite negative abdominal scans and other evidence to the contrary, she might have gallbladder disease without gallstones which he proved with a sophisticated radioactive tracer scan called an HIDA biliary study, which confirmed severe gallbladder dysfunction: the organ was removed by keyhole surgery, and since then she has never looked back.

DOCTORS DISSECTED

I immediately telephoned my patient to apologize. She was charming and replied that she felt lucky that a diagnosis had been made at last, and told me that all was forgiven as she now felt so well. She then apologised that she had been so rude when I had told her that she had depression. I was disarmed by her approach and said that apart from being very sorry, all I could do was go home and eat my hat. It is hard doing medicine but I forget at my peril that it is even harder being a patient.

Stomach ache and headache are among the most frequently presented conditions and with headaches I usually decide in the first 30 seconds if it is a headache that requires further investigations, as I will know if it is migraine in a matter of minutes. The patient inevitably will think they might have a brain tumour, so taking a history and examination is reassuring, although only one per cent of brain tumours present with a headache. More people present with 'tummy ache', that much used term even by adults, so reminiscent of childhood, than headache and that innocent phrase can be one of the most challenging diagnoses to make. There are two primary sorts of 'tummy ache', one that causes you to break out in sweat overnight and has a knife edged thrust to it and which demands immediate attention and then the sort which just goes on bubbling through your life. I will ask the patient whether the pain has ever woken them, or keeps them awake at night. I go on and on about how you must examine patients but in fact I do not believe you add much by your examination as a diagnosis is more likely to be in the history unless they have peritonitis. I always do an examination but history is more important and usually examination doesn't lend much to my intuitions, which by now are based on cumulative experience.

Women are easier to diagnose than men as men are shyer. Women's bodies, throughout their lives, are exposed to undressing more frequently but men are more difficult to examine, and it is easier to say to a woman, 'Slip your knickers off while I do a quick vaginal,' than to say to a man who may have prostate disease, 'Turn on your left side as I need to stick my finger up your anal canal.' Dr Stuttaford of *The Times* used to say, if you do the rectal, and it is surprising how reticent some doctors are, there is a little note up there with the diagnosis on it. I have hardly ever found anything with the exception of how the prostate feels, small or hard. This is an obvious example of the advantage of continuity of care undertaken by one doctor, because you will have notes, or even a latent memory of a particular patient's anatomy. There is little use to the examination if a different doctor undertakes it each year. I always say the prostate should feel as smooth as a squash ball with olive oil on it; if it feels like a wobbly walnut there is trouble. Smooth is the desirable texture, but not with nodules like a lentil that have been glued on with superglue – that is worrying.

This is the very week that in the *New England Journal of Medicine* (January 2013), there is the definitive statement regarding prostate illness that we should stop doing PSA blood testing in men for raised prostate antigens because this trusted stalwart of good practice, we are now being informed, does not save life and wastes financial resources. We have all been insisting on it being done annually for years and now telling our patients not to do it is going to be really, really difficult, because it is a complex set of arguments which end up demonstrating that a rectal examination is much more reliable but of course the examination is only as good as the person doing it. My female colleague says her finger is so short, because she is a slight build and she cannot get it up there high enough to have a proper feel but I have got a long-enough index finger. However, you have to know what you are doing, what you are looking for, how the prostate should feel when it is healthy and so on. So, the examination is only as reliable as the finger and the index of suspicion of the person doing it. You have got to be suspicious of anything irregular you feel – you have got to have the courage of your convictions and say, this is abnormal, but you have most importantly got to know what you are doing. This convincing research is a stunning volte-face, which has turned out to be the Emperor's New Clothes because it is 12 years that we have been doing PSAs and now the authorities tell us they will not save lives.

Yes, the clinical examination is unchanged although I hope that maybe now I take a better history, informed by so much more experience colouring my questions. I re-enter the room for a clinical examination including some aspects, which are not always relevant, taking the blood pressure for example as it will provide another chance to look at the patient from a general point of view as well as to focus on the symptom. If they are complaining of backache I pay attention as they recline on the couch as to their range of movement, power. Then follows the neurological examination despite the fact that I already know this is sciatica but not yet how much further investigation is required before I can advise a strategy. How they get on and off the couch is observed, all clues noted, and it is not a coincidence that we refer to a medical *investigation* because often the diagnosis will require similar skills to a detective.

Which reminds me both of a poignant experience of loss that happened almost 30 years ago and which was also the moment in time when a new and undiagnosed disease entered into my consulting room that was to change the course of both medical history and human civilization. Late in 1983 doctors became aware of patients dying of resistant types of pneumonia, occasionally in tandem with a type of skin cancer, which was known as Kaposi's sarcoma. It had been realized around 1982 in the USA that some of these individuals had an immune deficit caused by what was probably an infection: the pneumonia and other complications, such as rampant cytomegalovirus infection of the eye or gut being opportunistic rather than the primary problem. For a while the pathology of this remained obscure to us and I have an enduring memory of a long Easter Sunday lunch with friends, some of whom were medical, including the eminent dermatologist Richard Staughton and cardiologist Stephen Jenkins, in which we battled long and hard in conversation and argument about the possibilities of identifying the origins of this baffling new disease. Then, in May 1984, Dr. Robert Gallo identified a virus, which was named HTLV-III as the likely pathogen. This was a human retrovirus, one of a group of human T-lymphotropic viruses, which was subsequently re-named HIV in 1986.

It was in that year that we made the diagnosis of one of my long-standing patients, the actor Ian Charleson who was best known for his starring role as Olympic athlete Eric Liddell in the Oscar winning 1981 film *Chariots of Fire*. Four years later, Ian was to die under my care in his own home, in Hammersmith West London in 1990 at the age of 40. He had requested that as much publicity as possible should be given to the cause of his death – AIDS – so that the condition could be raised to greater public awareness, with his dying hope that of some of the prejudice and innuendo be abolished. Just before he died Charleson performed as Hamlet at the National Theatre with his face almost a mask and unrecognizably disfigured with the lesions of Kaposi's sarcoma. It was a remarkable performance, before he died a mere eight weeks after the end of the run that November. The Ian Charleson Day Centre, for those with HIV, is named in his memory.

I cannot deny that, over the years, one also dares to rely more on intuition. It may be during another consultation, or at four in the morning that someone will come into my mind that I saw the previous day and an alternative thought will pop up involuntarily. I wake up and write a note by my bed and return to check my notes the next day but only in the minority of occasions will my intuition lead me to call somebody back for further consultation. Your brain is still processing even though you have run on to the next patient, phone call, are having supper, or even when you are sleeping.

Years ago, the history and examination were the same but the outcome was different. Then, in regard to back pain, my only options would have been physiotherapy or painkillers or maybe a plain X-ray of the lumbar spine (I haven't ordered any of those for years); and wait, resting, yes, bed rest for six weeks. Now, I reach for my keyboard, print a request form for an MRI (Magnetic Resonance Imaging) scan, complete this in front of the patient for them to take away and make the appointment.

The post-modern world has evolved beyond expectation and now we can have instant access but then we just had our pagers. Now we have 4D ultrasound scanning in the office, and progressively have acquired CT scanning (an X-ray imaging technique), MRI, coronary artery bypass grafting, angioplasty and stents for narrowed or blocked arteries, opening the way for a multitude of minimal access surgical procedures that may be connected to critical conditions and diagnoses.

Despite that, these are not fundamental changes at all, as the GP is still a service professional, trained in the process of diagnosis and much of his time is spent on sorting out the trivia. There is an instant evaluation of the physiological, psychological, social and environmental status of each patient; the GP may then be the agent of referral to a specialist or to the laboratory, or to some other further investigation. None of that has altered in the three or more decades of my career but only the technical details of how, where and when. When there is no referral or investigation the pastoral role of the doctor becomes paramount to me, when intuition and subtle factors of judgement about what else might lie behind the symptoms, the psychosomatic aspect, must be judged and acted upon with a sensitivity which is hard to teach, but harder still to learn.

How does a doctor maintain this additional role without increasing dependency in his patients? There are more questions than answers here. What is more: can we afford the luxury of the holistic attitude in a system where the nation insists on the sacred cow – more a mythology than not – of free healthcare at the point of delivery? We must be realistic and with the population explosion since the inception of the NHS ask what can the nation afford in the way of primary care. One reason for the upsurge and deification of alternative or complementary medicine is that when patients opt to pay for homeopathy, osteopathy, acupuncture, or even astrologers and other deceivers what they are paying for, what they are seeking is quality time, a listening ear, care and sympathy from someone whom they believe to be professional, skilled, and committed to understanding the nature of their problem which is dismissed or at best regarded as unimportant, or trivial, by orthodox medicine.

Research has revealed in recent times two connected thoughts about general practice: one is that not only do patients value continuity of care above all else, but when it is provided by careful organization and deliberate strategy the outcomes for patients are better. No surprise there then, but why is it no longer a key part of the format of primary care? Why in our Health & Safety obsessed culture do we let something like continuity of care fade away? Second point: the nation extracts about 24 hours per week of patient contact time out of each GP while the other half of their time is spent in bureaucracy, administration and box-ticking of one sort or another, regardless of whether this is helpful or has even become necessary. It is criminal to waste clinical resources that have taken years of complex medical training to acquire, in this way.

In my early days in practice, a patient arrived who had just retired from his lifetime occupation as an engineer in Hong Kong where he had been involved in the inception and construction of the subway transport system. We spent an hour together documenting his history, when he first registered at the practice, at which time he told me about the time he had spent in a prisoner-of-war camp, tortured by the Japanese, during World War Two. Nearly 90 per cent of those incarcerated had died, and I was interested in what it was about him that had enabled his survival. He explained that as a boy he had been sent away to a harsh Jesuit boarding school in the North of England, telling me with a wry smile that the harshness of that experience fitted him out for anything. I too had been educated at the same school in Lancashire, as a result of which he and I had an implicit understanding.

He came back again for his winter 'flu injection 35 years after that first consultation. He had come by bus, from his home in south London to my clinic in Portobello Road, walking the last few hundred yards from the main road. He came up to my room on the first floor, and as he slipped off his jacket I remarked that it had been a year since I had seen him. I gave him the injection, and as he left he said, 'See you next year.' He is one hundred years old. Given his good state of health, he is on no medicines, what is his continuity of care all about? It is, at this point, that he knows that he does not have long to live and that I am there for him, whether the terminal event is a sudden stroke, or a heart attack, or a slower death if he should sustain an illness and that he trusts me to govern whatever will transpire to be his mortality which gives him comfort. Comfort to know that I am at the end of the phone for him 24/7.

In 1977, after I had completed some years as a postgraduate training for general practice, I spent some weeks in Rome working with a Professor of Cardiology. At midday we used to meet colleagues in the library for an aperitif, and then process through to the dining room, where we would sit at tables of four or six, for lunch. There were tablecloths, linen napkins, a typed menu: a starter of green salad maybe, then pasta, then a main course of fish or meat and then a piece of fruit, and coffee. How decadent you might say, although we went back to the clinics or wards by 2 pm after heated arguments about patients, discussions about any problems and maybe a phone call or three, perhaps a letter or two dictated and a lot of chit-chat about love, politics, football.

These days I hit the office before 7 am to the relentless cascade of e-mails. My morning continues with me seeing patients from 7.30 am to 1 pm and then it is a hasty apple or two at the desk while reading the post, followed by house calls, the hospital, and more consultations at the surgery. In the evening, after packing up at 7 pm I have to turn my attention to all the things we have to do to keep up for our professional appraisal, re-validation and re-licensing: the rituals of postgraduate study and improvement, the compulsory gathering of points for 'CPD' (continuing professional development).

A study from Israel has looked at eight judges and followed their judgements on applications made by prisoners to parole boards. It was revealed that at the beginning of the working day the judges granted two-thirds of the applications, but as the hours passed, fewer and fewer. After each of the meal breaks the number increased again. Why do the judges appear to lack balanced judgement? It looks as if a low blood sugar is important – how much time has passed since a meal – plus how many cases they have been presiding over: how bored they are. It appears that even judges are biased by human factors. Maybe we medics, under great pressure for 'productivity', should think about this, for the sake of our patients and their welfare. The essence of good care may well be careful communication but the essence of that continues to be clarity, thought, time, and trust. And in an era when personal care by GPs is 'under the cosh', with cutbacks and the pressures of burgeoning red tape (despite the promises of Mr Cameron's government) none of that comes easy. It does seem that I spend a lot of time seething and grumbling about the state of things, in a state of bolshie dissent. But, Hippocratic Oath and all that, my only interest is in doing what is best for my patients and yet, in a world where the NHS GP is also an independent subcontractor, our monopoly employer, Her Majesty's Government, has an over-riding imperative: saving money. But boiling over with frustration about such matters does not always occupy my mind: often I find myself marvelling at the sometimes extraordinary and often delightful things that happen to a general practitioner.

Late one summer afternoon, I was sitting in my consulting room, back to the window, talking to my last patient of the day. Behind me I heard the familiar sound of the window cleaner's ladder against the outside balcony, and became aware that he had arrived at my first floor window. Suddenly, the sash was raised and he stuck his head in, over my shoulder, saying, 'Hello, sir.' The patient stood up and seized the window cleaner by the hand, beaming, a look of pleasure and astonishment on his face. Tom Windows as we called him, had been his rear gunner, in a Lancaster bomber, the patient being an NCO who, despite his lack of officer status had been a pilot and both had survived the conflict. This was their first meeting for many years, and there was only one thing for it: we all sauntered down to the Ladbroke Arms to celebrate with a Guinness, me thinking, 'This is a moment I shall remember.'

11
PAIN HAS
AN ELEMENT OF BLANK

Illness is the doctor to whom we pay most heed; to kindness, to knowledge, we make promise only; pain we obey.

Marcel Proust

Martin, it is no secret that we both suffer chronically from dysfunctional disorders, which have no reliable 'cure'. Migraine has chased you throughout your life and I live with a feral creature, or serpentine enemy, in my bowel, irritable bowel syndrome (IBS), which tries to create havoc with my life. As you have often told me we are not going to die from our pains but neither is there any guaranteed treatment or cure to be found in orthodox medicine, or anywhere come to that. Both of these conditions are examples that many GPs find among the most challenging to manage. For many patients there is no successful treatment outcome, so they are often relegated to being thought of as those 'heart-sink' patients that GPs come to dread finding waiting for them on a Monday morning. I thought it might be helpful if we were together to deconstruct some of our own subjective thoughts about their insistent presence, which have been significantly demoralizing to both of our lives.

While I feel that you couldn't say that either of us has chosen our specialties you have got to ask the question, even if we cannot answer it as to whether what we do as professionals, our daily exposure to other people's pain and suffering, and its involuntary impact on our bodies makes those conditions worse.

PAIN HAS AN ELEMENT OF BLANK

Let's begin by you telling me about your migraine, and as a psychotherapist maybe I shall have a different way of listening to you, so tell me what you first remember about your migraines.

When I was a boy I remember that I had a thing that in earlier history was referred to as acidosis. I only know this through personal reflection and I have never discussed it with my parents, but more recently it has been called periodic syndrome, nothing to do with menstrual periods, and when you diagnose children with it we are told that it is a condition suffered by intelligent children with demanding parents. Usually, I got it when I was about to leave for school. You might go green and then it gets worse at school and you have to go home, but I went away to boarding school at nine and there you just had to pull yourself together. To begin with it was abdominal pain with vomiting and by about mid-afternoon I was usually better and everyone thought that I had been swinging a leg but it wasn't like that at all and I had it in the holidays too when I had to be put to bed with the curtains shut. I first had it in 1953 when my father took me to Billy Smart's Circus on a bit of green grass at Totteridge Lane. I remember we were sitting on wooden benches and I started to be sick and we missed the circus and that is a classic example of what often also happens with migraine where you often look forward to something hugely, like getting on an aeroplane to fly away, or Christmas morning and you are struck down with adult migraine and the illness ruins everything for you and often for others too. I first started getting the headaches along with vomiting at nine or 10 and my parents thought it was to do with butter and then later my father got me some stuff called Cafergot, which was caffeine and ergotamine which you had to crunch up, like a Smartie. I don't remember having headaches again until I was 16 when along with A-levels they returned and by the time I was a medical student the headaches

231

were really bad, classic migraine, and I was irritable with noise. In those days I could get rid of them by going to sleep, but not now, not as I got older. Even small amounts of alcohol have become a trigger.

Do you get visual disturbances with them?

No, I've never had 'fortification spectrum' as it is called.

Catherine wheels, I call mine.

Catherine wheels? No. Well, the classification is called 'migraine with aura and migraine without aura' and mine is without and I might or might not be sick.

It was interesting that the other morning, I have never had it before but I woke up and felt for some moments that I was in a different world, everything seemed to be silent except I could hear bells chiming in the distance, but there were no bells to be heard when I listened and then I went downstairs and the visuals all started to firework in my eyes but fortunately no headache followed.

Yes, an aura and they can come in many other ways; some people may smell bacon frying. People also talk about whether there is a mood change, which presages it, and so if I am quite high tonight it may mean a migraine is on its way. I am quite cyclothymic anyway and mostly my mood is a bit high rather than a bit low, so I cannot really tell but when I'm recovering from one I also get high but I'm not sure if that's just from relief that the bloody thing has gone.

PAIN HAS AN ELEMENT OF BLANK

How do they manifest now? Have they got worse as you have got older?

The pain has got worse – it is in my left eye and I cannot work through the pain any more and noise exacerbates it – I cannot think with it, or to put it differently, trying to think makes it hurt more.

Well, you are high powered, fast moving and almost manically driven to pack as much as possible into every hour, both pleasure and work, do you think it could be your body's way of telling you something, enforcing rest and isolation?

When I had a sabbatical year I thought it might go away but it was exactly the same, except when I was motorcycling in Australia. Now, I have to strategize myself in order not to miss out on the good things in life and so I always have a triptan tablet in my pocket, or I may even take one in advance as a precaution, but the problem is not taking too many tablets as there can be a rebound problem when it wears off and you then end up with another migraine the next day.

Is it worse at any particular time of day?

Yes, it is usually between 3 and 4 in the morning when the pain wakes me and it takes me ages – like minutes – to force myself out of bed and deal with the awful pain and find a tablet which gets rid of it in an hour. If I didn't take the triptan it would be there all day and I wouldn't be able to work.

You refer to the triptan medication as your talisman but it can be addictive so how much professional help have you sought for migraine?

Just to clarify about the medication – if you take triptan it will switch them off immediately – but the other milder drugs like propranolol and those things seem to have stopped working for me.

Who is responsible for your medication?

Myself. I have only ever once gone for formal treatment two years ago when I went to the National Hospital for Neurology at Queen's Square to see a Dr Matharu, otherwise I have self medicated. The triptans came out in 1992 and before that there was no treatment except for the Cafergot, which I had as a boy, which is dangerous; it is not a safe drug to use.

Didn't your father know it had dangerous side effects?

Well, he was an anaesthetist and he wasn't much good at that sort of thing, but he still insisted on medicating us; we didn't have a GP once we were older.

You have prescribed triptans for yourself?

Yes, and arrogant enough to think I know a bit more about it than most doctors because suffering from it you sort of feel you are better informed.

PAIN HAS AN ELEMENT OF BLANK

What do you know about it?

Well I know all the options for treatment; I didn't think I could learn anything but I did learn something from Dr Matharu, finally.

When patients consult you is it easier for you, than medics who are non-sufferers, to be sure it is migraine and not something more sinister?

Having read about it and followed the research, I think I'm quite good and I know all about the different sorts of migraine. A young girl came today because her face now goes numb on the left with migraine but it didn't use to. I explained to her, 'There are different sorts and now you have this other type.'

How did you know it was not a brain tumour?

That is why she came, she was afraid of that, but I've seen people who cannot lift their arm up with a migraine, but the paralysis has gone the next day. Unlike a tumour it doesn't last – a tumour doesn't go away, the symptom persists. Migraine is like your IBS – there is a whole hotchpotch of symptoms and they can all change over time.

OK, let's go back to why you gave in and went to consult Dr Matharu at the National Hospital?

I realized I was getting worse and I had become addicted to the triptans, I was keeping a migraine diary, and found out that I was getting more than 16 headaches a month. I thought some of my headaches must be rebound headaches caused by the triptans and I must come off them. There is a book called *Headache in Clinical Practice* by Peter Goadsby who is Australian and one of the world migraine wizards but he has now moved to UCLA. Not so good with patients but a brilliant researcher and lecturer, I've heard him and was really impressed with him. I rang Queen's Square but he had left and so I went along to see Dr Matharu instead, just as an ordinary punter, and I had to fill in a huge questionnaire, just like doing an exam. I went to his private migraine clinic. He is a very nice man and the first thing I learnt was that he has got migraine and the next thing was that my own diagnosis was evident to him as being correct without doing scans, etc. He could see how knowledgeable I was but he was not at all happy and said, 'You are addicted to the triptans and you have to stop. There are two ways, the easy and the hard way. The easy way is to come into hospital for two weeks and it will be terrible and the hard way is to do it on your own.' I thought I couldn't take two weeks off work, impossible, how will they cope without me? He also said, 'You have to drink enough water, take exercise, go to sleep at the same time every day, not over sleep, not under sleep, no alcohol.' Well, that doesn't fit very well with being the sort of 24/7 general practitioner. It fits in better with being a civil servant and going home on the 6.20 to Purley.

He was serious?

Absolutely. No humour at all. I paid lip service to what he said and kept a good migraine diary and I didn't take more than two triptans a week. I started by taking two days off work and taking no meds and having a pretty rotten time. Oh! He also told me I should take riboflavin, that is vitamin B2, and coenzyme Q10, but he said none of the preventions would work, 'Because you are an addict.'

PAIN HAS AN ELEMENT OF BLANK

Are you now off triptans?

Well, I have had two already this week, and where are we? Oh, it's Tuesday. Well, I haven't had one yet today, but I am much better than I was.

But you took two triptans yesterday.

Yes, but this is an unusual time, we are incandescent at work and two doctors down and I was down with the rotavirus and have had to drag myself back to work as nobody was free to do my back-up for me, so I am on my back foot, but that is fine.

To what degree has migraine impacted on your life?

Oh, it's been an absolutely dominant theme, just as my sex life – my love life, if you like – acts as a steel rail running along, the other steel rail that the train runs on is my migraine. More dominant than food, the clothes I wear, more dominant than anything. It stops you being cocky and first of all it makes you more aware of clinical medicine. There is no test for migraine, there is only the story, just as with clinical depression, well there is no test for IBS either but there the diagnosis is critically to be found in what has been screened for and what can then be excluded. Loads of people do go and see a neurologist because they are so frightened and they want a brain scan.

I do not go along with the idea that there is a meticulous, self-punishing, migraine personality, but I have noticed quite often some other doctors are suffering from appalling headaches, often of course made worse by drinking, and they don't get it that they are suffering from migraine. Doctors are supposed not to get ill.

237

I never thought I would catch the rotavirus but then I did. I think as a group we are quite blind to the stress we are under – we attempt and fail to deal with it in our professional development groups, through our faulty relationships, and through alcohol, oh lots of faulty ways. I have had to learn to control my drinking even though I love a gin and tonic but lots of doctors do not. I think they are pretty useless at taking any disciplined care of their health.

Pain is so difficult to measure objectively, so how would you measure your migraines?

For me it is a boring pain, it bores into me and post-operative pain is nothing compared to a migraine. When I had a laparotomy I woke up the next day with a migraine but I had this drip in my arm, something up my nose and the nurses refused to give me a tablet for my migraine – they insisted I wait for the anaesthetist. Eventually, he arrived and I said, 'I am in awful pain.' He replied, 'No, you are nil-by-mouth,' but the post-operative pain was nothing by comparison and the lesson you learn is always to have one triptan tablet in your bedside drawer.

I mentioned earlier that I have suffered too from migraine but not incapacitating like yours, and mine are always prefaced by visual disturbance and not necessarily followed by any pain. On the whole they don't disturb my life because I know the visual disturbance will only last for 20 minutes, but if it carried on I would be terrified it might never stop. In fact, if I knew it would definitely end I would quite enjoy the firework display of Catherine wheels. Because I am not plagued by bad headaches or nausea they don't affect my life like my IBS. The most

interesting, or rather disturbing migraine I have ever had was after my son was born. It had been a very difficult pregnancy with a high forceps birth and as soon as I knew I had a boy I was in conflict about whether to circumcise him or not. I couldn't bear the thought, but knew my mother would not talk to me again if I didn't. Anyway, the nurse gave him to me and I got a blinding migraine; I couldn't hold him, which turned out to presage a terrible experience of an extended postnatal depression.

You remember me saying an hour ago that there is a correlation between migraine and depression and 60 per cent of people with chronic migraine need treatment for depression at some stage. I am sure there is another relationship between chronic migraine and neuro-endocrinology, and your story embodies it. Quite a lot of women get headaches when they secrete prolactin from their pituitary, which means when they start breast-feeding they may get a lot of headaches, and when you were handed the baby you may have had a rush of prolactin. I am wondering if on being handed your son you walloped out some prolactin, switched on your migraine and set light to the whole process of postnatal depression.

If 60 per cent suffer from depression what about you?

I don't think I have ever suffered from depression, I have been blue about things but that is different from the illness. I am interested about when you described taking Alex into your arms and getting PND because I think there is, I keep going back to the word neuroendocrine, a definite link with endocrinology. I am talking about neurotransmitters and the subtleties of those things, and I am interested to think about their links with your

239

IBS and my migraine because we now know the intestines are the second brain and my migraines started, as I have explained with something like juvenile IBS. I have often said that kids who also experienced my earliest symptoms will often grow into migraineurs, or they will have IBS.

I am wondering how you diagnose IBS in your patients, and whether it can only be through the exclusion tests?

There are two groups really: there are those who have never been appraised and they come along because of their symptoms and talk about bloating, or pain or both and then you are going to take a history and make a consultant referral if they have never been examined. Often the women will also be at the constipation end of the spectrum.

Are men more likely to have diarrhoea?

Well, that is my impression, I don't know what the research shows but I don't know many men who complain about constipation and if they do I am likely to think that it may be sinister.

But my experience is that men spend much more time in the loo, on the loo, than women do.

Do they?

Yes, all women will tell you that.

PAIN HAS AN ELEMENT OF BLANK

Well, I always think it a bit odd that people have books and things in the loo and maybe some men do, but I wouldn't make that generalization and if a man has constipation I have a very low threshold for sending him off for a sigmoidoscopy, if not a colonoscopy. I saw a man today of 38 who has had rectal bleeding which is not caused by piles and I immediately sent him off. 'If you were 28 I wouldn't be doing this but you are just getting up into the age group.'* It is very unusual for women to complain of rectal bleeding at that age unless they have piles caused through pregnancy. There is another group who come along, who have been told they have IBS but have never been investigated by a previous GP. They have erroneously been told to have a high-fibre diet, or take Fybogel, or something and now and again, after proper screening you discover that one of them has Crohn's disease, or coeliac disease. IBS is interesting, it is like back ache, which when you take a proper interest in it, it becomes interesting because you have got to think of all the possibilities and now and again you hit a coconut – you pick up something serious – you are glad that you did the tests. I know you are phobic about being scoped but you do know there are 'virtual' colonoscopies, which are not invasive, don't you? I have had both procedures and I thought the virtual was pretty good, as it only takes 35 seconds but you still have to have something shoved up your bum, but then you do with the barium enema you finally succumbed to.

The thing with me is that it is all in the mind, the fantasy. When I am forced to succumb to becoming a patient I am a very good patient, and there is no problem at all. I have such a vivid and active imagination, which can be destructive, and helpfully I am able to recognize the same factor in some of my clients

---

* This young man turned out on investigation to have an aggressive intestinal tumour, which had to be surgically removed and he has since been treated by chemotherapy.

241

who develop phobias. I just heard you say you have had both kinds of colonoscopy yourself and now I am wondering why? We started off talking about your migraines but now we seem to have discovered that we both suffer from migraine and IBS although with opposite quantities of pain. Migraine doesn't curtail my life whereas IBS does. I hate it, it eats into my life and I feel I am always making a Faustian pact. I promise not to eat anything that I like ever again in return for a few pain free days a week, although that is no guarantee either. It is only the fact that there are some days that are pain free, which keeps me from falling into a very deep despair. I have noticed that you have made a few referrals to interventions regarding your own bowel that sound as if they turned out not to be IBS related and which I am now curious about. IBS seems to me to be all about *opinions*, which are packaged with an amazing diversity of theory and an absence of proof. Tell me, if you will, about your abdominal pains. We have talked about your migraines but in the past when persuading me to be investigated, you indicated that you have also consulted for abdominal pain although you never elucidated the context.

I had recurrent abdominal pain – not only as a child, but as an adult. I started having it in my forties and then I had one bout in the night, which was bad enough for me to call my colleague who had to come over and give me a pethidine injection. That was an awful bout of pain and I thought I might have an intestinal obstruction and then I thought, 'Don't be silly, don't be neurotic, it is just spastic colon or IBS.' I have always had a slight degree of IBS and quite variable bowel habits, with the occasional shits. Also, whenever I got mouth ulcers I got a sore bum and I thought this was some funny variant but then I would ignore all that. When I had my sabbatical I thought it would all go away, that was the year 2000, but then I had a second bad attack, and I thought as soon as I find the time to, I will do something about it. I came back from my travels and went to see Prof Silk who insisted I be properly investigated. 'You are 50 and you must have a colonoscopy and a CT scan and every investigation going.'

He did all the tests and when Professor Bartram the radiologist had finished a blooming long barium X-ray I said, 'What do you think?' He retorted, 'Everything is normal.' I went back to Silk who said, 'Have you seen your barium studies? They are the most abnormal I have ever seen. I think you have got an internal hernia and a bit of your intestine is poking through into a hole in your peritoneum and into the space where your kidney used to be and you are intermittently obstructing your small bowel. That is what the X-ray looks like to me. You will now need a laparoscopy.'

So why did Bartram say it was a normal bowel?

I said exactly that and Silk said, 'Oh, he always says that to people; he doesn't like engaging in any conversation – he is the radiologist!' I was referred for a keyhole look straight through my tummy button to see what was obstructing my small intestine and the consultant said, 'You do realize that if I find an abnormality I cannot deal with through the laparoscopy I will have to cut you up, so do you want me to wake you up first, or to do it?' I told him to just to get on and do it, just to do it. 'Okay, but you might wake up with an ileostomy, or a colostomy.' I replied that I didn't care, too bad and just to get on and do whatever was necessary there and then.

Oh, my god.

DOCTORS DISSECTED

I woke up cut open and I have a scar all the way down here. [So do I, from belly to pubis!] I asked what the diagnosis was and he replied, 'You had a congenital malrotation of the duodenum with fibrous bands which have been contracting over the years and which have obstructed your small bowel.' It was a congenital abnormality, which had slowly worsened, and by the time I was 50 it had declared its hand. He said 'We have aligned your duodenum as it ought to be and snipped all the fibrous bands and stuck it all back together.' I just went home after five or six days and hung about a bit and on the fourteenth day I started erecting my pergola at Green Farm, I thought this will make me better, and it did. Since then I have only had one bout of that pain, it did not need an injection but it was bad enough to make me vomit. I don't know what that was about. There is a lot of abdominal scarring that gets concealed under the label of IBS, because too many doctors will just assume it is more of the same rather than fully investigate a new symptom. You need to have quite a high temperature, to be really ill, before they will believe it is something different. A bit of a flight of ideas here but have you heard of faecal transplants?

No.

This is a new development in medicine where they take faeces from someone who is well and whisk them around in a Magi-mix or something, filter the mix with a sieve and shove it into someone suffering from IBS. Yes it is true, it has been done a lot but mostly in America and this is orthodoxy and not something New Age. They put the mixture into your small intestine, but not as an enema. You do not have to drink it as it is passed into the intestine through a nasogastric tube. They put the tube all the way down through your stomach and into your small intestine

244

and then run the liquid in, about a pint of it, and it is being used in the treatment of Crohn's disease too, but mainly in IBS, with quite good outcomes. It is like giving somebody probiotics but instead you are giving them someone else's healthy faecal organisms.

But why, why not use a probiotic like Symprove?

Because these are friendly organisms and your bowel is probably full of unfriendly ones; you have somehow got a colony of bad ones and probiotics are just one colony of one type of bacteria and this way it is the full panoply. In fact I am trying to find someone in London who can do it as I have got a young girl with very, very bad IBS.

People get such bad, bad IBS. It can be the same with migraine and in that spectrum there are still even much worse sufferers than you.

Exactly and people will do anything to try and escape the pain, and they are having things implanted in their brains, little electrodes, little batteries under their skin because there are people whose lives are ruined by both of these conditions.

Yes, and I'm probably in the upper middle with my IBS.

Yes, and if the scale is out of ten then I would place you, at a guess, at 6.5 − 7.

Well done, exactly where I would place myself.

The same with my migraine, but this girl's IBS all started on her gap year in South America where she was admitted to hospital with dysentery. That has all been cured now, the tests are negative but her IBS is a post-infection one. She was fine before she got ill so I think she is a candidate for a faecal transplant because she has got the wrong bugs inside of her.

She doesn't feel disgusted?

Well, everyone who hears about it feels disgusted and I do not like the idea of it much myself, but they do purify it a bit and they sieve out all the bits of carrot and stuff – yes, it is a bit of a noxious idea.

Are we not back to methods used in Ancient Greece and are there not pictures of 18th-century physicians encouraging patients to drink their urine? I think historically urine has been used both as a dental bleach and antiseptic. In the 'Egyptian Book of the Dead' Spell 165 is a prohibition to protect the dead from eating their faeces in the after world, in the absence of food.

I think that was a bit mad.

I was talking to someone the other day about our book whose father was a very experienced GP practising 40 years ago and the subject of faecal transplants came up. She told me that he used to say that as soon as somebody sat down in front of him, if he let his mind go blank, he could tell if somebody had cancer just by his or her smell. He thought that until the end of

PAIN HAS AN ELEMENT OF BLANK

World War Two human beings still operated with some of their animal nature, from which, with the 'aid' of technology we have now become entirely removed. When scanners were still non-existent, doctors had to depend far more on their senses and for example on the variable smells of faeces and urine in order to inform their diagnoses, in the same way that the police depend on their sniffer dogs to trace drug traffic. Perhaps more relevant is the fact that the earliest Egyptian physicians, according to the Kahun medical papyrus, would describe a gynaecological ailment as having the smell of 'burned meat'.

Martin, I also want to share with you some of the observations that our mutual colleague and friend, Matt Banks, expressed in a conversation with me about IBS because they resonate with and illuminate some of the things you have explained.*

Matt – I was intrigued after I referred to you a young man suffering from chronic IBS, to hear that you explained to him that no specialist understood more than about 20 per cent of the human gut.

Hmm, I am not sure where I got that figure from but it was only meant as an anecdotal perspective. I suppose it takes into account a sort of global knowledge of how little we can offer our IBS patients. It represents both our medical ignorance and our limited ability to understand physiological, or pathological processes going on inside of the bowel and also the absence of effective treatments that we can offer. We can also only identify very few of the bacteria in the bowel. Nobody knows the precise figure but the understanding is that we only know 10 to 30 per cent of the bacteria present. There is so much to understand, and

---

* Matt is Consultant Gastroenterologist at University College London Hospital NHS Trust.

even with understanding, the medications that we have are not particularly effective at changing the abnormalities of many of the bowel's neurological pathways.

When you talk about medications, I find that the worst thing about having IBS is the way the bowel is the most recalcitrant of organs in its response to drugs. Nothing makes any difference to my pain and that is what I find so frustrating, not even strong doses of codeine, not antidepressants like amitriptyline,* nothing at all whereas if you have a headache you can take something and it tends to pass.

Yes, the bowel is obstinate and I have to agree that I have little faith in any of the recommended medicines, although very occasionally I do use antidepressant drugs like amitryptiline and even the Prozac family of SSRIs, but as you say their impact on visceral pain is very different from limb pain, or even chronic headaches.

I have suffered from IBS for many years but it definitely got progressively worse after I had major although benign pelvic surgery about 12 years ago. My GP told me after I started complaining of increased pain that he thought a bowel that had been submitted to pelvic surgery would typically cause a lot more problems than a 'virgin' bowel. I cannot help thinking that the bowel, or its yards of intestine, were not designed to be dragged out into the light of day and then stuffed back into the abdomen but when I finally went to see a particularly arrogant but renowned consultant whose specialty is in IBS he told me

---

*   Also used for chronic and unexplained pain control.

that I was talking a lot of nonsense, and that my hypothesis was mythology-speak that had nothing to do with physiology!

Well, how do you answer that? [LONG PAUSE] From my personal experience I have had so many patients who have developed IBS after major surgery and I think it is fairly common, even after an appendicectomy. Just because no measurement in physiology before and after surgery has been done, as far as I know, does not mean it does not happen, but only that from a purely scientific point of view it is unexplained and unproven. Whether it is mythology or not, you cannot ignore abdominal symptoms and just because you cannot equate those symptoms with a measurable change in physiology it simply does not mean they don't exist and are mythical; therefore I think his argument is flawed. From an observational point of view when you take the bowel out and resection it and zip someone up it doesn't anyhow begin to work again for a few days and there is a sigh of relief when it does. I think that is a very good demonstration of an observable sequence of events taking place in the bowel and yes it recovers but does it ever fully recover? I don't think it does. At the same time IBS is very unlikely ever to do you any severe anatomic harm.

I think that IBS develops over a sequence of events and some of the studies that have been published are flawed but there is a very nice study in Canada where slurry from a local farm overflowed and went into the local water supply and a large proportion of the local population went down with an e.coli gastroenteritis. The researchers followed all those patients up and a large number developed IBS after they had recovered from the serious illness. Many of those patients had had IBS symptoms before but they just increased in magnitude and of the patients who developed more chronic symptoms, 20 per cent of them never recovered their former health. I think again that demonstrates that the bowel doesn't often recover well from trauma. The potential of the bowel to recover well depends on other factors.

Whether genetics plays a role I don't know, but IBS tends to be quite common in family clusters and again whether that may be due to genetics as well as environmental factors, or solely environmental factors, I still don't know. I think there are triggers and I think there are presupposing factors.

I believe, and there is mounting evidence, that a large proportion of the abnormal physiology in IBS is abnormal pain processing that is taking place within the bowel wall itself. There is some evidence to suggest that in the models that can be measured chronic anxiety alters the way those nerves function. It is a little bit more complex than that because once those messages have left the bowel they are then processed in your spine. If you can imagine you have nerves, or hairs however you want to imagine, within the bowel wall which will respond to so many features like stretch and tension, fluid consistency, temperature change and many other influences which can affect the ways the bowel contracts and stretches – for example, the amount of gas in the bowel, the degree of fermentation, the acid component, the alkaline component which depends upon the degree of bacterial fermentation, and the bacteria which create the environment. That environment depends on how quickly the bowel is contracting and how quickly things get through; there are so many unpredictable factors. Ultimately, pain will be more likely to occur if those nerves are being irritated by anything on that list, which then send messages from the bowel to the bottom of the spine, which make their way up the spinal cord and then meet the synapses and the primitive brain where those messages are processed into your conscious brain. All of those multiple pathways may be affected in IBS, we just don't yet know which, but we do know that it is at the beginning of the journey from the bowel that those nerves are probably affected. That is the reason that neurogastroenterology is fast becoming an important new sub-division for us to understand.

PAIN HAS AN ELEMENT OF BLANK

And how long is that journey?

Less than a second. A lot of your pain is, I think, down to abnormalities of pathways and one of the most likely influences is going to be chronic anxiety levels, but how that happens we just don't yet know. My colleague, Anton Emmanuel who is at both University College Hospital and the National Hospital for Neurology, considers that if you can manage those abnormal pathways at the very beginning of the process then you will have a greater chance of reducing symptoms.

Would you describe yourself as a neurogastroenterologist?

No, not really because what I am describing is not just neurological as there are so many other pathways involved although my Ph.D was on neurophysiology. I did spend four years just studying the physiology of the bowel, so in a sense I am, yes I suppose I am a neurogastroenterologist. Yes, that is what I am.

I am interested to know why you chose Gastroenterology as your specialty?

I think it was because after I qualified as a junior doctor, I was drawn to the unknown and the breadth of the subject, which although it wasn't in its infancy when I went into it in 1995, it was only just starting to grow. Parallels at the time were Cardiology but the heart felt very finite to me, it really did, it felt too small, which is also why I didn't go into surgery.

I think you previously told me that when you were a boy you were interested in the subterranean, the ocean and you thought you might become a marine biologist so not all together a surprising change of direction, your professional commitment to the unfathomable depths of the gut.

Yes, I wanted and still want to be intellectually challenged. There is also a procedural component to my work in terms of diagnosis; I enjoy the delicate manual finesse of endoscopy. Being a surgeon would have limited me primarily to cutting up the body and not understanding the patient or their condition.

We have, for obvious reasons been focusing on IBS but I am aware that in your working day you are often divided between trying to divine the mysteries of IBS, or the concreteness of making cancer diagnoses. I cannot imagine there are two more mutually exclusive conditions.

Depending on their severity, some cancers may be curable with very little intervention, and then you look at a patient with severe and debilitating IBS and very little can be done about it. I don't know which is the better evil, really.

How do you set about in deciding how to proceed with your diagnosis?

Most of the time I will have made a preliminary diagnosis within a few minutes of the person sitting in front of me, and examining them makes very little difference to my diagnosis, which must sound arrogant. However, I do carry out a physical examination because the patients feel reassured when they are examined and it allows me more time to get the feel of their personalities. Normally, the examination just corroborates my assessment and allows the patient to feel cared about. Yes, within minutes the history of IBS is usually such that I have excluded major organic disease.

It seems that as far back as the commentaries in the medical papyri of the ancient Egyptians the palpation of the body has had a symbolic as well as practical importance, which made it possible for the physician in addition to diagnosis, to both reassure and even to heal by the laying on of his hands.

If you had to choose between organic disease of the bowel and IBS, which I know is silly...

I would probably choose...[LONG PAUSE]...I don't know, but if it were me I would probably choose IBS simply because on an individual level – although you cannot control your bowel physiology – at least you can feel as if you doing as much as you can. One of the problems with cancers is there is always that uncertainty, the unknown, of how it will turn out.

We are back to the unknown.

We are, aren't we, but even the earliest cancer may have metastasized and you just do not know, nobody does, not until five more years, post diagnosis, of waiting has passed. There is not a single one of the existing tests that can predict what will happen within the subsequent five years post diagnosis. No test is fallible, so that uncertainty in my private life would be harder for me to live with. At least with IBS you know that some days it is going to get worse and other days it is going to get better. For some their IBS comes on predictably at 4 in the afternoon, and you know it is not going to kill you, not directly.

When I talk to the GPs most of them fear making mistakes with patients with abdominal pain more than those complaining of headaches.

Yes, because the pelvis is a huge space and catastrophic mistakes are easily made which results in carrying out far more investigations than you may want to do which in itself can compound people's anxiety that there may be something seriously wrong with them. If someone like you comes with a 10-year history of a symptom then it is highly unlikely to be a malignancy, but it is always difficult to take the risk of not investigating fully.

I am sure the degree of pain that I suffer with would have killed me if it were anything other than IBS. Of course I also know that having IBS doesn't mean that I won't develop cancer as well at some future time. I will never forget attending a weekly course in Mindfulness with a close friend. Beforehand, we would meet in Carlucci's every week and I would lament that I couldn't eat anything and that my colon was in spasm and then she started to complain of what at first was a tiny nagging pain, nothing like the intensity of mine. After a few weeks I persuaded her to see my doctor and within a year she was dead from pancreatic cancer, which all started with an almost undetectable murmur of discomfort.

Has your microscopic involvement with the bowel day in and out had any impact on your personal life?

PAIN HAS AN ELEMENT OF BLANK

Interestingly, I have developed mild IBS, which doesn't bother me too much, but now my oldest daughter, who is 13, also seems to have developed it.

You have developed mild IBS?

I think so.

You mean you haven't gone through your own exclusion processes of diagnosis?

No. No, I haven't but I think many people develop mild IBS at some stage in their lives but they either are not aware of it, don't admit it, ignore it, or are too embarrassed to admit it. I had a very stable family upbringing – although possibly lacking in communication skills – I remember going through periods when I was very anxious as a young boy and I did have tummy-ache from time to time. I never really thought about it until recently. Lots of children get tummy-ache and now I wonder whether mine was more or less than normal. I recently asked my mother and she thought mine might have been a little bit worse than my brother's.

There is a little piece of research currently being done about looking back as to whether people who develop IBS also had symptoms as children and it seems to be a little more common. Perhaps those early trigger influences were there from quite early on. I think I got anxious as a child but about all quite normal things like homework and exams, so now I don't know whether my professional awareness has resulted in me becoming hypervigilant, if you will, and that has started to generate symptoms of its own. I do think hypervigilance plays a powerful part and perhaps even compounds the problem, but I am not sure, and I certainly don't think there has been transference from me to my daughter.

I also suffer from lower back pain which I have had on and off, better now, but I have had years of quite bad back pain and I've got a slipped disc but at my age people's discs become worn out and bulge anyway.

At your age Matt…but also you are a fanatical sportsman and also, if I can interrupt, when you talk about homework and exams I bet, no I know you were a perfectionist with very high and self imposed standards to maintain!

Yes, at 45 the disc is definitely sticking out a bit, but at my age it is normal for the spine to start to deteriorate. I don't know whether my back pain is related to my bowel or not but a lot of my IBS patients have considerable back pain as well. I am also probably hypervigilant about my family's bowel habits but I hope I manage it very subtly. I don't mention it to them, but privately I hope things are happening normally. I suppose I have a fear that they might develop one of the illnesses that I am dealing with because I am aware and surrounded by them the whole of my time. Childhood Crohn's, for example, worries me – it is such an awful disease in children, which always has a horrible course, it is so debilitating. I suppose I have a deep fear of my family becoming ill but I tend to focus on the bowel, it is crazy I know, but then as a family we have experienced premature life-threatening illness, so perhaps it is understandable too.

No, it is not at all crazy but it doesn't make your life any easier. I have learnt several things from our conversation and much of what you say knowledgeably elucidates Martin's spontaneous observations.

PAIN HAS AN ELEMENT OF BLANK

With relevance to myself I have to admit that, for various childhood reasons, as well as adult trauma coming into the mix, I would score 100 per cent for hypervigilance, so perhaps you have divulged the cause if not the cure. It is the events of my life and not neurosis that has caused the vigilance and all I can do, having tried everything from hypnotherapy, through medication, to yoga is to endure my Pilgrim's burden and try to let go of the pain.

After talking to Matt it made me feel the hopelessness, or limits of medicine even more strongly. I feel like a warrior fighting chronic pain, not surrendering, not letting the serpent shut down my life with its impossible demands and prohibitions. As long as it doesn't stop me from working, as that is my personal benchmark of pain, whether or not I can work through it, and whether in spite of its bite I can still be a celebrant of life.

It also struck me as an involuntary thought that the bowel is the most creative of the body's organs. Blood comes in different types and also with different markers, but in health it remains constant, as do all the organs generally. By contrast, even a healthy bowel is capable of producing a vast canvas of different textures, colours, shapes forms, along with a compendium of sounds and scales of smells for the gut is very much an autonomous living organ with a stubborn mind of its own. The variety of organisms peacefully (at times) co-existing within our gut are said to number more than the planets in a galaxy, and the gut will continue to function even after we are brain dead. Yet, paradoxically, the influence from the brain both positive and negative has been shown to be symptomatically and functionally profoundly significant. Gut bacteria produce hundreds of neurotransmitters, which are used by the body to regulate learning, memory and mood. Gut bacteria are also known to produce up to 95 per cent of the body's supply of serotonin, which is a contributor to feelings of well-being and happiness. What a piece of work is a man!

Once I had this thought about its chameleon and obstinate nature it made it easier for me to understand why so many creative and often powerful people have become preoccupied by, or suffered with, their bowel and its produce. The list is endless and predominantly male but it includes that master of scatology, Rabelais, Luther, Samuel Pepys, Swift, de Sade, Freud, Darwin, Proust, Hitler, Gandhi, Beckett, and Dr John Harvey Kellogg. Kurt Cobain curiously wrote in his suicide note, 'I thank you all from the pit of my burning nauseous stomach.' While Oliver Cromwell wrote to the synod, 'I beseech you in the bowels of Christ think it possible you may be mistaken.'

12
CATCHING UP WITH COSMO (JUNE 2012)

There has been two years' distance in time since my first meeting with Cosmo, which is due to an uncanny happening when Martin saved my life. For a substantial period after this incident I developed acute writer's block that put the completion of our book in jeopardy.

It was June 2011. I was on holiday with my husband John at our Provençal house, perched on a hill, which overlooks medieval ramparts, where Martin and his partner Rachel had joined us for a few days to relax and work on our book. We sat down to dinner as the sun was setting and divine house martins were dive-bombing across the water. Rachel had cooked lamb with couscous, and the table was candlelit. Martin was sitting beside me on a rustic wooden bench, Rachel was directly opposite and John was sitting opposite Martin. I became aware that I had swallowed badly and that something, maybe no more than a grain, had uncomfortably lodged in my throat, but to my surprise I was unable to cough, or even to clear my throat. I had been rendered dumb in one instant. The conversation was animated and nobody seemed to notice that I had lost the ability to speak, or to draw attention to myself. To begin with I was only focused on the internal flush of shame I experience when physical things feel out of control.

Quickly, I became aware that not only could I not draw breath but that I didn't seem able to move and that I now had only the weird sensation of moving outside of and above myself and hovering mute above my head; I was drowning except there wasn't any water. It felt as though I was suffocating on my breath and without my being able to signal that I was now paralyzed and in real danger. Outside of my orbit and in the distant room, I now heard Rachel ask if I was all right, but I was no longer there. I tried to shake my head and lift my hand. I can remember a calm inner coherence as mute, I spoke only to myself, 'There is no time left for them to call the emergency *pompiers* but you are sitting beside one of the most skilled doctors in the world, if he cannot save you then you must allow yourself to die, to float away.' I was unfathomably calm. I was not flying, I was no longer drowning; I was floating along with those swallows towards infinity.

Martin seemed to be beside me and behind me, and I was almost limp when I heard his characteristic 'Hey!' There was an almighty punch as he grabbed me into the Heimlich maneuver and began deep abdominal thrusts. My breath returned, Martin checked me for internal bruising and sat down. Rachel was tearful and my husband – the eternal optimist – had returned to his seat and not without a faint bewilderment continued his meal. Nobody said anything more and the meal continued.

All that night, high on the hill and cortisol, I lay outside beside the reflecting water surface in the company of the shooting stars, fireflies and waxing moon. The next morning Martin told me that he had also found it difficult to sleep and that unusually for him he had woken 'teary' with thoughts of how it might all have ended differently around that candle-lit dinner table on our deserted hilltop.

There was an unexpected and disturbing long-term consequence to the event: while my breath had returned I now found myself unable to write, or to think about another sentence, or even an interview for a year.

Cosmo, tell me what you have been doing since we last met – I think you are now at Charing Cross Hospital, and also are still working as a volunteer for the Ambulance Service? Your dad proudly pulled a newspaper cutting out of his wallet about you being first on the scene, informally and out of hours, at a dramatic motorway accident. I know how busy you are as it has been impossible to pin you down for months and I have only persisted because Martin reassured me that it was not so much due to a reluctance to come back and continue our conversation, but rather that you have just finished a punishing cycle of night duty.

I was offered a place as Senior House Officer at Charing Cross and I've been there for almost a year. I'm doing anaesthetics training, although I haven't yet done any anaesthetics because at the moment I'm combining a Critical Care specialist training with it, so I've added an extra training year while I combine Accident and Emergency with Acute Medicine and hence my lack of availability.

Despite being so lean, you are a bit greedy Cosmo, filling your satchel with so many qualifications. How long will it be now before you do an unsupervised anaesthetic?

I have three months where I have always got someone senior very close beside and effectively dedicated to teaching me. For the first few weeks the consultant is right there but after that induction they might then be around in the next room doing some paperwork. After three months you have an assessment and if you make the grade they sign you off as having a basic competency level and then you can conduct your own patient lists, with another senior anaesthetist close by.

It must be an extraordinary moment when you first put someone to sleep? Such a weird colloquial term...

I have already been doing it as a trainee, just getting unofficial experience but always with someone beside me. It gets scary when you find yourself out there all on your own.

Oh, you sound like you are out at sea. Perhaps even scarier is the moment when you have to wake the patient up.

I think that is probably true. Yes, that is true and lots of people don't realize that it is actually more dangerous waking somebody up than putting them to sleep – well, sometimes. People can have problems when they are waking up in terms of breathing issues and every anaesthetist does it in a slightly different way; every patient reacts differently in terms of how quickly they recover and in terms of what faculties they regain first, which can be quite difficult to predict. Every anaesthetist has to have their recipe if you like.

What period of time do you stay with the patient in Recovery?

It depends on the kind of operation, how unstable they are, what drugs you had to give them and how long they will take to recover and how rocky the road is as they are waking up. On simple cases you may only stay 10 minutes or so, and then leave them in Recovery but with others it can be a lot longer.

How long?

Well, I don't really know much about it yet, but some of them go to Intensive Care where it can be a matter of days, which is a prolonged and controlled waking up that depends on what has being happening. Days to wait, depending on how unstable the patient is.

It strikes me that it is possibly the most mysterious aspect of medicine.

Yeah, we don't have a great understanding of how the drugs work, of what they really do, because we still don't understand the brain particularly well. I think that is why it is hard to understand anaesthetic drugs, when we don't even know quite what the brain is doing when it is not awake and what the neurological differences are between sleeping and waking.

Do you think as a subgroup anaesthetists tend to be obsessional?

I think we tend to be controlling. I've never seen a survey but it would be interesting, as there seem to be two types. There are powerful and high achieving girls who are often very controlling. There are lots of them, probably more than boys, because it is a very good job for women. The work/life time balance works with families but you also need to be focused and to multitask. There are lots of girls who are very clever; they are the really clever ones of the medical school lot, the sharp ones, who can see exactly what is happening. Some of the guys are quite controlling and can also be a bit obsessive but then there are others who like the excitement angle and the rest of the time are more relaxed. They often enjoy using all the drugs that most doctors wouldn't be comfortable touching. You get some anaesthetists who are very chilled out but I don't know if that's because they are very confident in what they are doing, 'Give a little bit more of this and a bit more of that.' It may be that they are so confident that they can even relax a bit.

Where do you fit in?

I'm quite obsessive-compulsive disordered in some ways. When I revise I have to have all my notes neatly sorted and like Dad, I like my things being in the right place. When I write my notes I always have the same structure about how I put plans into place. I think people have told me before that I like things being done my way, so I'm probably fairly controlling.

Yes, your dad likes things in their place; he doesn't like food spilt on the table, or anything dropped on to the floor. He is precise and tidy.

Yes, Dad is tidy, but in other ways I can be chaotic. I am quite good at set tasks, at going through them in a sensible manner so that I have a structure but when I have to multitask, or go into flurries of activities, then I get into chaos and everything is at the back of my head, muddled up. No, I'm not continuously obsessive.

CATCHING UP WITH COSMO (JUNE 2012)

Is there any clinical situation in the last year – out of hundreds of patients – that leaps out of your memory?

Most I forget, but there was a lady from Vietnam, I think she was 92, and she came in with a very bad pneumonia, and accompanied by her family. No, it was only her son, there was just the two of them, and she was likely going to die and he knew that and he was devastated. All the nurses found it hard, he was so attached to her – well, perhaps she was only 75, I'm struggling to remember, no, as he must have been about 65. It didn't affect me so much but the nurses were talking about it, how her son held her hand all night and wept.

That account is about the way the nurses felt, but what about something where you were affected.

I cannot think of anything immediately. I haven't had many young deaths, which would be different but I haven't had that, as it has always been elderly people who have died.

Try to think about something relating to you.

I've got nothing that pops out...I had another lady who came in with really bad pneumonia. I see so much pneumonia, it is massive and one of the largest causes of death every year, and there are so many strains about. There are many conditions that are worse illnesses than those people usually think of. It is all about medical PR. Lots of people are terrified of HIV although people are now living with the virus for 30 years, but it doesn't stop people being terrified of it, even though I think most are over the stigma. Heterosexual HIV is a more common cause now, but it is not a bad diagnosis to have compared with other things. Cancer is not a good diagnosis but it has also got lots of mortality statistics going for it but if you have a diagnosis of heart failure, depending on its severity, that can be much, much more dangerous than any cancer diagnosis, and, depending on the severity, with a much higher mortality and burden on your life, but nobody talks with such terror about heart failure as they do about cancer.

Perhaps the treatment isn't as frightening, but you have moved away from the personal!

Heart failure can be pretty bad and then emphysema is again a worse diagnosis but it is funny isn't it, what scares people. Oh, I see lots of pneumonia and the recovery all depends on your immune system and general health. With young people they are often in and out as they have bigger reserves and are without any additional chronic illness, because it is a disease that affects you when you are frail. I did have a young guy at Hillingdon Hospital with a terrible pneumonia and he had to go to Intensive Care and have a machine breathe for him for a week. It was scary as it was very, very severe. He made a full recovery. Yes, he wrote a card to our ward, so that was reassuring – to see him admitted so sick and then recovered.

Oh, I have just got a contract with the London Ambulance Service, outside of my hospital work, so I now have a non-paid job with them and the insurance conditions are different and I can actually work and treat people on the ambulance and not just observe. I had a dream recently that I was first at a car crash, but I can't remember a lot about it now although I was thinking a lot about the dream the day after. I should have written it down. I think I was the first to get to the accident but there was conflict between the ambulance response team and me. Yes, Dr Cosmo Scurr, was first on the scene, but the crew didn't want me to be involved. I was on the motorway but then we were suddenly treating the patients in a cave. I woke up and thought that it was real.

Dreams are 'real'. Were you negotiating the contract when you had the dream?

Yes, that's possible.

The dream could reflect that but also I have just realized, quite literally, that is what the newspaper cutting your father showed to me, where you were first on the scene, was about. Symbolically, the dream might also reflect the fact that while you are on a high-speed career trajectory with its reputation for high technology, your unconscious has drawn your attention to the dark and primitive areas of caveman knowledge about the way the brain functions and consciousness.

The other day I heard an item on the news about kidneys, which made me think of you. I think the statistic was that one kidney is sold every hour somewhere in the world for transplant purposes and it made me think about you and your brother Ben, who I know has recently had a transplant. There seems to be such demand for kidneys for transplant.

I think it is the most common major organ transplant that is performed, probably because other transplants, unlike kidneys, cannot be done from live donors. In addition, each cadaver provides two kidneys and also there are people with kidney failure already being kept alive on dialysis. Yes, there are many people living and waiting for a kidney transplant, unlike with heart-transplant patients, who often die before a heart becomes available. Even so, kidney disease is not a common disorder in comparison with heart failure, lung disease and pneumonia, of which there are enormous numbers. The problem with kidneys is that there is still reluctance from the public to join the organ donation register.

Scotland has new legislation; I think that was the basis of the news item.

No, it is Wales and I think it is only slightly but not massively helpful. What I find interesting is that in all decisions about your health care as an adult no family member can make a decision on your behalf and even if you are incapacitated, even if you have dementia, the people looking after you, the doctors will discuss with your family as to what you would have wanted, and that takes place at a holistic level. The doctors try to find out your beliefs, whether you would want a medical intervention, but your family cannot make that decision for you. A family can say 'No,' or 'I don't want him to have an op to fix this,' but the medical team will say, 'It is what he wants, or would have wanted.' They will ask if there might be a paper trail with the GP. In contrast, after death even if the individual says, 'I want to give my organs, I want to donate my organs,' then the next of kin will have the final say and can even protest, 'My loved one has already been through too much invasive medicine so, no!' That is a very interesting anomaly: in your life only you can make the decisions but after death, as soon as you die, it is the next of kin who get the say.

It must have been tough for you getting to your wedding in Norway and then discovering that Ben had arrived in a relative state of undiagnosed kidney failure, and that despite his

reputation for wit and fun he had lost the twinkle in his eyes when he made your wedding toast. I think Martin told me that he was admitted to hospital immediately on his return to the UK and that fortunately his partner's blood group was compatible and he was able to donate Ben a kidney. It was impossible for me to find out how Ben was doing from Martin because even with the help of Google I couldn't always decipher his Latin penned terminology. I am not an idiot but that is how Martin tends to deal with painful things and feelings. He speaks scientifically. I imagine it must have been very hard for you discovering that Ben was so unwell and is now acutely suffering from a disease with which you potentially share its trajectory.

Yeah. Exactly. Absolutely. Ben has had a tough time. It gave him quite a shock; it gave us all quite a shock.

All? But it gave you a personal shock too, didn't it?

Yeah, but we don't know how much of it is kidney disease and how much is the diabetes affecting his kidney. Ben has been dealt a hard blow by having both the kidney disease and the diabetes and that makes it a bit easier for me because I don't have the diabetes, which makes it less stressful to witness. I don't have to think, 'I am next,' although it is true that I will be 'next' at some point. So…

And Ben did have a transplant didn't he, but as I understood, or misunderstood it from Martin, it was rejected.

No, it has worked but he has got some problems with it. We are now not sure if it is antibody problems or autoimmune disease affecting the new kidney. They are actually a bit similar. It is an immune reaction so he has had to have this extra treatment to dampen down the antibodies and to clean his blood from antibodies, which has been quite a hard procedure for him.

Do you find it hard to be close to him watching both similarities and differences, but significant similarities?

You mean in terms of the disease? Don't think so. No, it's just difficult for me to get the time off work to go along to his consultations with him, which I can't do. I try to be free and we talk about it on the phone but to be honest some of it is even over my head as it is very specific and unusual, it's a very niche area of medicine. I think it's over my dad's head too, not to mention we are getting the information second hand from Ben. It is complicated stuff that only the consultants dealing with it, only those very specific kidney consultants, not even all kidney consultants understand. Yes it is very niche. Ben is trying to tell it all to us and we are trying to interpret it but I think the truth is really we don't have a clue what is actually going on and that is quite difficult. Going along to the appointments with him would be the best thing to do, but I often cannot take the time off work to do it.

Has any of this changed your attitude to your own health? I remember hearing from Martin that you gave everyone a shock recently when you had some acute and mysterious heart-related episode.

When was that?

CATCHING UP WITH COSMO (JUNE 2012)

Well, I didn't expect you to remember it. You can't remember?

When was that?

Well, it was in the last few months, it was before your wedding and you had to call for an emergency ambulance.

Oh, yes, that was really weird, that was odd, and I actually had to ask Cecilie to call an ambulance for me. Oh, I felt very strange indeed about calling an ambulance.

You did eventually recognize that you were ill?

Yeah. It is just that my heart was going mad, and I was sitting there reading a book and I felt very strange and clammy and faint. I was sitting there counting my pulse just to see what it was doing and it was all very odd. It was going very irregularly and then very fast. I had noted it first in the morning when it had been doing a few irregular beats and then pausing, then doing a few more irregular beats and pausing and then going back to normal. I thought it was absolutely fine. I ignored it and it was fine all day but then in the evening it started going quite fast and pausing and then going faster and then beating very, very fast.

What is fast?

It was going at 160 beats a minute. Young people can get this thing when their heart goes into fast rhythms and you have to have some medicine to stop it doing that, but I felt so odd and unusually ill and dizzy and I wanted to get an ECG to see what

271

it was doing so we had to call an ambulance…my heart kept changing its rhythm.

Were you satisfied with the ambulance?

Yeah, and they took me to my own hospital, Charing Cross, because it was the nearest and that was strange too. I ended up in Casualty, which everyone found hysterical and the staff started making jokes about me being on a stretcher.

The other thing I have to be careful about is that, if you have kidney disease, you can have this problem with the salts in your body and that can make your heart do dangerous things. I was thinking in the back of my head, 'Oh God, maybe my kidneys have gone a bit off and that's why my heart is doing funny things…I really do have to go to hospital and get my bloods checked as well.' So yeah, it was strange.

Frightening, I imagine for Cecilie to see you go off in an ambulance.

Yes, I think it must have been, and I think it must have given her a bit of a shock because I sat there for a while in the chair, monitoring it without saying anything to her at all. I hadn't told her, I hadn't wanted to worry her about the morning episodes and then suddenly all I said was, 'You need to call me an ambulance now.'

Oh, heavens with nothing in between, how awful for her.

She is a worrier and I didn't want to worry her when it would have been fine if it had just settled down and she wouldn't have needed to be worried by what was going on.

CATCHING UP WITH COSMO (JUNE 2012)

Did she come to hospital with you?

Yeah, we went along and luckily everything was okay so it was quite funny. But I still don't know what it was. I do drink a lot of coffee, which I suppose I drink to keep going, so I have had cut down a lot on caffeine.

And in general has it made you more careful about your health? Or are you still disinclined to monitor your blood?

I still haven't had a follow-up, but I did have my bloods done in Emergency and my creatinine levels were not too bad, just a tiny bit higher than they were when we last talked, but it is quite hard to monitor your kidney functioning because of the way it works. It can go off the page just like that, it doesn't linearly deteriorate. The blood tests don't get worse to begin with but then at some point they go off the radar. The blood tests are not a huge marker. So, no, not really, I'm still working just as hard every minute of the day and often the night as well.

You are so driven at work, so greedy for experience. How does that affect Cecilie, seeing you work so hard?

I don't think it is easy for her and I did cut back an extra shift the other day because even I thought it was ridiculous.

Do you want to have children?

Yes, I think so, but I don't know how you fit them in, though.

Stop doing all these extra things but that would be quite a compromise for you. Why do you need to do all the extramural ambulance stuff when you already have such a punishing training schedule?

It is quite good for me career wise, for the stuff I want to do later, when you need to have both medical and paramedical skills. I want to work both in and out of hospital. It is like working with the ambulance service except I want to work within the Helicopter Emergency Medical Service (HEMS). It is competitive because there are so few jobs, yes, it is very, very competitive, and that's why I have to do extra things. You have to be able to bring something special to the selection table when the time comes.

Yes, it is very, very competitive as there are so few anaesthetists working like that, hardly any even at the Royal London Hospital, which is the HEMS centre. There are only two who do it as part of their job plan and a couple of others who help out but their main job is in the hospital and a couple more posts out of London.

Your devotion to the NHS and your training is so evident and I wonder what you feel about colleagues – in their next decade – who have become consultants and then decide that the NHS burns them out. They often complain about the necessity of compromising their clinical excellence for bureaucracy and management. In the doctors' group I run – where the remit is to talk about us and not about our patients, to talk about feelings, but you would have no time for that. A couple of the doctors, one is a paediatrician, and the other a psychiatrist at Chelsea both feel so frustrated with the NHS, frustrated that so much money has been invested in their trainings but now they feel that the bureaucracy of the service is responsible for them not being able to maximize their

clinical skills. The paediatrician says that it's not unusual for him to have to give up clinics to go on a 'fire drill day', or to do a special course in how to lift patients, which frustrates him and makes his clinics shorter and even less efficient and satisfactory to run. Now, he has had enough of being controlled in a service, which he believes can only function clinically effectively if the controls are removed from the managers and returned to the clinicians but he says this will never happen, so he wants out. I don't think it is primarily about the money to be made in the private sector, but a deep disillusionment, which drains the NHS work of personal satisfaction for many of its most skilled clinicians.

There are a few aspects here, and in terms of wanting to look after your patients well, it is always going to be a matter of how much time you have. Dad can choose to give a patient half an hour, or even an hour if they need it, or even want it, if they can afford to pay for it, and in the NHS you will get six minutes. Of course you will look after your patient better if you are a general practitioner, or private consultant with all that time. The problem is that it all comes down to whom is it that you want to serve and what you want to get out of your job. Everyone needs health care, everyone needs to be looked after and there is only so much money and only so many doctors and that is why GPs only have six minutes but they are not sitting around doing nothing the rest of the time. We would all like more time to look after our patients. It would be easier and you could do more, and when you do more you get more job satisfaction because the patient in front of you feels better because they have had more of your time, so you feel good. It is quite common that people say, 'I want more time and I cannot look after my patients properly in the NHS so I am leaving.' But who is that really for? They are not really doing it for the patient. It is for them.

If they feel they cannot look after their patients or, worse still, are putting lives at unnecessary risk because of a lack of time…

No, sorry, but it is still for them; the patients who cannot afford private practice will still only get six minutes. People say that in a noble way, which sounds like they are doing it for the patients but they are doing it for themselves.

But isn't your self the most important person in terms of focusing on integrity?

True, but you have to be honest. These guys who are leaving the NHS can still do it better than their juniors can, even if they only have six minutes. There are two facets here: do you jump ship, and if you do jump ship you don't do it to make it better for the patient. You have made it worse for them because, by leaving, there is now less experience in the NHS. You don't do it to make things better for the patients, to look after them properly, because you are now doing it for different people who can afford to pay for your time, which is also fine so long as you are honest about it. To answer the second part of the question: if you stay in the NHS is there too much time wasted on management and non-clinical time? Yes, you do have to go on these courses but there are a few more issues here. For example does any doctor only work their contracted hours? In lots of jobs people don't only work their contracted hours, and in medicine most people don't and they never did in the past. If you are really worried about looking after your patients, then your clinic can go on longer. It is up to you. Many clinics do go on longer because people are trying to do the best for their patients and after clinic hours you will dictate your letters in your own time, and some of the consultants will even go back and do ward rounds after their clinics. It is true that not all

276

do that in my experience, but they could if they wanted to do so.

When you talk about it being a waste of time sending doctors on lifting courses well you have to remember we now live in a litigious society. I don't really blame employers for trying to protect themselves against being sued for injury at work. It is easy for us to get annoyed at the managers but in the past organizations have been heavily stung by tribunals for not being covered, because they have not trained people in Health and Safety. I agree that these trainings are all rubbish, or do I? Actually, if someone has a cardiac arrest, or falls as they are getting on to the table, then consultants may well have to bend down and lift people. Did you recently read about that footballer that had the cardiac arrest on the pitch and a consultant rushed on and saved him? I was talking to a resuscitation training officer who explained to me how every few years all the NHS consultants have to do a course in CPR, and this consultant had protested and said, 'I don't do cardiopulmonary resuscitation, I am a consultant.' Six weeks later he ran into action on the football pitch but he had had to be forced on to that course by bureaucracy, but perhaps one day it might be relevant to all of us.

I think that is why both Martin and Dr Peter Holden speaking on the BBC after the terrorist attack, think there is now too much specialization in medical trainings. Now you are explaining that there have to be additional courses for procedures which their trainings historically provided for automatically, and which seem to return into the foreground of memory when there is an emergency. Can you not see that there may be a process of disillusion and burn out in your own world?

I think Private Practice can be a good thing because it relieves the resources of the NHS and it allows people to have a higher quality of care if they want and can afford it. It is a free country and we should be allowed to use our money as we like. Anyhow, there is the revenue and it all goes back into the system in terms of taxes but I find it a bit rich when my colleagues come across as noble, when it is not for the patient, it is just a personal choice. I don't think medicine is a noble or altruistic choice. I do it because I am interested, reasonably paid, it is a quite fun job and I enjoy it. I enjoy being paid well and if I wanted to I would still consult a private consultant. I think these people who are opting out are kidding themselves: they are doing it for themselves and not for the patient. I don't criticize the choice, it is a fine choice, but they shouldn't claim that it is 'for the patients'.

When your dad read our other interview he said, 'Gosh, I learnt more than I've ever known about Cosmo's thoughts and memories and feelings through reading about him.' Neither of you like to show your feelings too much. It seems you both need to hang on to your composure; you don't like to communicate directly, intimately about difficult things. Well, in particular feelings, which can, like surgery or dissection, be quite messy.

We are both English and cut from the same stone.

You are not cut from exactly the same stone, as there is also your mother. I know something about your dad's family but all I know about your mother is that she is very different. I am told she is extraverted, charismatic and presumably good at communicating her feelings.

Well, she is extraverted and silly but I wouldn't say she is particularly good at communicating about personal things. I don't think any of us are very good at it. She is not brilliant at holding a conversation either, because she gets very easily distracted; she is silly but she is very good fun. We all tend to be a bit superficial in the family. Mum is eccentric, very energetic professionally and outgoing but people can be like that without you really knowing much about them. It is just another defence mechanism at work isn't it? Mum might say, 'How was your day?' Then, without a pause the next question is, 'What shall we have for dinner?' She is quite scatty, so that makes it hard to have a serious conversation with her, which with the combination of Dad is probably why I am not at all trained in that area. But lots of doctors tend to be like that and they tend to laugh a lot, or tell a lot of jokes, or speak a lot in a blurting sort of embarrassed way. Well, I am quite odd most of the time, bizarre and I spend most of my time at work making jokes.

Oh, to the patients or the staff?

Sometimes to the patients, but definitely to the staff.

When you arrived on that ambulance trolley, you made a joke?

Yes, just childish things like when the first nurse turned up to look after me I said, 'Why do I get the rubbish nurse?' Silly things like that. They know you don't think that but it is kind of continuous like that at work. The gallows humour, which keeps it fun.

It keeps it light.

Yes, and that is important for me! But if I go to the theatre, or read then I prefer sad stories, sad films and darkness.

Does that provide you with an acceptable outlet to be sentimental?

Yes, I do get sentimental sometimes. I like sad music, but I do like fun as well, although I like quite heavy stuff, and definitely sad films where I like a sad ending rather than a happy ending. I like dark things. I liked the novel *The Secret History*, about those students where things go wrong, and I like true books. I don't read that much fiction. I like to read something where, at the end of it, I feel like I've learnt something concrete. I read quite a lot of pseudo-medical things and historical things about war and revisioned history. I like watching factual stuff about people. I'm meeting a friend of mine when I leave you who is an officer in Afghanistan and we like talking about what he has seen in his life, the trauma and how it makes him feel.

He has probably seen a lot of death too.

Yeah, and of young people too, which I haven't seen. Yes, of children. He has found it very hard being non-medical, and feeling helpless and having dying Afghan children brought to him about which he couldn't do anything, which is very sad.

Do you think of your dad as being proud of you?

Yes, I think so but he gets a bit mixed up with what I am doing but then what I am doing is often a bit odd.

13

THE MEANING
OF LIFE IS LIFE

Dr Mansur Ahmad FRCS worked in the NHS running his own GP practice from 1970 until he retired from the NHS at the age of 68 since when he has been working in part-time private practice.

Mansur, please will you tell me how you came to be a doctor.

I will tell you how it began. I passed my Matriculation [equivalent to O-levels here] in Pakistan in 1948, just after Partition. The desire to be a doctor was truly a deep feeling that happened inside of me. My family was in the engineering business, we had a factory during the Second World War. The factory was making objects, such as cigarette cases, basic cutlery, Primus stoves and metal covers for syringes for the British army.

I had no medical background. I used to have stomach upsets, and go regularly to see the local doctor for advice but, somehow, his treatment did not clear up my symptoms. When I did my O-levels, I thought to myself, 'Why cannot I also become a doctor and sort out my tummy?' Most important too was the fact that I was the eldest son and expected to look after the family. We had a big family, which consisted of parents, grandfather and six siblings, so I had all the responsibility. My father and grandfather wanted me to work in an office but I said, 'I want to become a doctor.' It was just my spontaneous wish, and I am telling you the true story. I went to Murray College in Sialkot, which was a Christian college where the principal came from Scotland. At that time the entry to medical school was through the merit of the A-levels and in the provincial

281

list of students who passed I was around number 30. The highest band was sent to King Edward Medical College in Lahore that has a long history of excellence from the days of the British Empire and I got my place there. At that time I was 17.

The thing is, I have been a bookworm since my childhood, and my parents were very protective of me and they did not want me to mix with the children who were not studious enough. I used to read all the newspapers, and I knew everything about the Second World War, and I still know everything by heart. I knew everything about the atom bomb and the American intervention after Pearl Harbour. I came first in my first and second year's MBBS [Bachelor of Medicine exam], but afterwards – when I went on to study pathology – my rank came down a little but I did pass in my time and I did my first house job in ENT [ears nose and throat] when I used to see cases of diphtheria but we had no vaccines at that time and I had to do daily, emergency tracheotomies for breathing. I used to do all that very early on my career and I was already quite at ease.

I remember one thing from my childhood. In 1936 my auntie passed away and everybody was weeping and on that evening I felt very unwell and my parents took me to the Christian Mission Hospital in Sialkot to have my throat examined. The lady doctor there came from Holland and we had to wait a long time to see her but I shall never forget her smiling face, like an angel. Honestly, I shall never forget that face, even now you can see my eyes have become a little watery. She examined me and saw that there were white membranes over my tonsils and then she gave me diphtheria antibodies serum and that injection saved me and I am still here and that is my true story. So, when I became a doctor I learnt a lot about ENT during the year working in hospital and after that I joined the Government Service and I went out to the villages on a horse carrying a bag with a few unsophisticated drugs but after only one year, most unfortunately, my father passed away in 1960 at the age of 53.

THE MEANING OF LIFE IS LIFE

He had a rheumatic heart and as a young doctor I looked after him and I saw that his heart was enlarged and there was a loud murmur too. He developed pulmonary hypertension and I gave him mercurial diuretics. I read all the books to find out how to look after him. In those days the only medicines available for heart diseases were mercurial diuretics and the plant Digitalis but the crucial thing to know is there is also a loss of potassium and at that age I was not knowledgeable enough to know how to replace his potassium. One evening I was giving him his milk and he just passed away. My auntie also died from a rheumatic heart and she used to take Digitalis mixture. The rheumatic heart was very common and they used to say, 'It licks the joints and bites the heart,' because there is mitral-valve damage.

Now I had a big financial burden to look after my family and I said to myself, 'I have to do something more than simple rural medicine.' By chance, I read an advert that the primary Fellowship to the Royal College of Surgeons course was being started for the first time outside of England, in Lahore, and I applied for it. Because I had been a good medical student I was accepted and they took about 70 doctors. I started to study and, although I was married with one child, I locked myself into the student hostel for six months and I told my wife she must stay with my mother. For those six months, I was just reading and shut up quite alone in that room. I sent for all the latest literature and I read and read and I passed the exam. They only passed 20 of us, but somehow I did it. Then I got a training job in Mayo Hospital as Registrar in Surgery in preparation for coming to the UK, which I had to do to get Part Two of the FRCS. I got a scholarship from the Commonwealth and came here with my wife Greta who is English. My first job was in Scotland at the Royal Infirmary, Dundee where I worked in Casualty to get my General Medical Council registration. After that I worked in different hospitals around the country and then I moved to Harefield Hospital, where I joined them as Cardiothoracic Registrar in 1967. I had passed my Part Two FRCS in 1966 in Glasgow.

Did you find any prejudice in your English colleagues?

Long before I came to the UK my grandfather was an Anglophile, he was illiterate but he knew everything about British history and he always used to tell me how the British rule had improved India. He was an ordinary person but his values and thinking became part of my mindset too and I was prepared to put up with any initial difficulties. However, I did experience some inevitable prejudice when I first set up on my own in general practice in Harrow. I started with a small list of 600 patients and 250 of them immediately left. I understood that they might have felt insecure coming to a foreign and coloured doctor. I knew that patients were human and that they often feel exceptionally helpless when they are taken ill and that it is difficult to shake off ideas that have been built up over many years, but I did not let that defeat me, as you will find out.

Did your grandfather also die of heart disease?

No, he died at the age of 100 but as a young person he had suffered many infections, including plague: he lost one eye and he survived the plague. Grandfather had only two children as my grandmother had died from postnatal bleeding and my grandfather raised my dad and my aunt as a single parent. He worked hard and said, 'I will look after my children.' He used to tell me that if there were an accident on the roadside, a local person may or may not stop to help but an English priest will always stop his car and come to help.

THE MEANING OF LIFE IS LIFE

Was your grandfather a Muslim?

Yes, but he was not a radical. He was, in my words, a passionate humanist, he believed in humanity and how to be passionate about a fellow human being and that is what I learnt from him. And then my mother, she always used to tell me, 'Do not worry about your pain, please think about the other person's pain.' She was also illiterate but these two things I have never forgotten, which gave me the empathetic context when I became a doctor, to think about the other person's pain and I still remember my mum's words.

Was it difficult for you being a Pakistani immigrant to England in the early 1960s.

No. When I came, there was no immigration problem so almost everybody looked at me in a happy way and with a smile, as there were not many immigrants here. My English wife, Greta took me to Belgium and Holland for a holiday where an elderly person took his hat off and welcomed me to Holland because things were not at all bad. It was only after Idi Amin and the Ugandan upheaval that Ted Heath had to start the refugee camps and all that, then it became too much. I still think the most tolerant country in this world is Britain.

Ah! Holland. It sounds as if you were at Harefield Hospital at a very exciting time.

Yes, in 1968 I became Senior Registrar in Cardiothoracic Surgery at Harefield and I used to work with Magdi Yacoub doing all the major cardiac operations. After open-heart surgery, one of our team had to stay with the patient and measure their potassium levels every two or three hours.

So your hypothesis about your father was right.

At that time in Harefield, Magdi Yacoub started doing his first coronary artery bypass and that was the beginning of coronary artery bypass surgery and I was present. Then we used mitral valves [prosthetic and hetero/homografts] for mitral-valve replacement and of course I thought sadly of my dad and wished I could have helped him, but in 1960 there was no mitral valve replacement. To begin with we saw so many cases of rheumatic heart disease but since 1970 onwards there has been a huge decrease in its incidence because general health has improved and it is now a disease of the past. In 1970 I could have applied for a consultant's job but I thought then I might have to move my family to Scotland, or the North of England, so I decided to avoid the hassle and settle down in general practice.

We lived in Carpenders Park and I got a job, a partnership with two English doctors in Harrow. When I joined in 1970 we had four branch surgeries and we had a rota and after one year I took over one of the branch surgeries. I separated from my partners in a happy way and started my own two-room surgery. I received half the list of another retired doctor in the area and then my practice flourished and by '78 or '79 my list went up to four thousand. Normally, a single handed GP cannot have more than 3,500 patients. So I can say in a humble way, I was a good doctor. I knew that the biggest problem in general practice is not to miss a diagnosis. Some mistakes are bound to happen but overall I have not missed much and over the years one gains so much experience to avoid making mistakes. The personal liking between the patient and the doctor is an important factor, regardless of whether the doctor is English or Asian. The initial contact is very personal. I believe that as soon as the patient enters the room, in the first 40 or so seconds, they form an opinion of whether they like the doctor behind the desk. Of course the doctor does the same thing but he has to try to be even in his responses. The eye contact tells you so much. I think if you listen to the patient and respect what they are saying to you then they are going to be more hopeful of receiving your sympathetic attention.

In 1970 I had only two rooms, and no secretary or receptionist, and I had to open the door to the patients, write all the repeat prescriptions, which I used to leave outside in a box, and also the referrals when I used to write the information for the patient on a letterhead paper and give it to them to take it to the hospital and make an appointment. Since then the changes that have taken place in the bureaucracy of general practice are phenomenal, from simple letters by hand, now we have to do it by electronic referrals [Choose and Book] and the last government spent one billion pounds on the software, which is faulty.

What did it feel like for you going from a cutting edge hospital to a small surgery?

Hospital work goes on at 70 miles an hour and general practice at 20. I have enjoyed being able to see my patients over a long period of time. General practice is a holistic branch of medicine, where we should aim to cover the person as a whole. When I began as a GP, the ethos of British family practice used to be that a whole family knew you; sometimes they even received you into their home as a family member. When I became a GP, in 1970, people came with their families and then they brought along their wives and their children and the continuity of care was in action and the past history of my patients was in my head. But today's practice of ten-minute consultations (and often lack of continuity of care) is not enough time to absorb enough information about patients who are strangers to you. Hospital medicine is organ based but in general practice you treat the person in a bio/psycho/social holistic context. I remember in 1968 I attended a lecture given by Dame Cicely Saunders at the Royal College of GPs and she started her talk, which I will never forget, with the observation that pain has three aspects and it can be physical, psychological or social, as a single item or in combination. I have never forgotten her words that whoever comes to see you is in pain and you must listen to them with respect and never reject them and now that is my golden rule too.

How does a doctor work on that principle now?

It is not possible to do so, but it is what I learnt and my daughter is a doctor too now and I told her, 'Please make sure you always treat the patient in an empathic way.' Whatever I would do for myself when I am in pain, I will do the same for a patient and I want her to do the same for her patients. In this case you cannot go wrong and most of the rules of the GMC are covered by this one sentence, 'Treat the patient as you would like to be treated yourself.' You do not need to read 20 books, you just have to remember your responsibility to attend to whatever problem the patient brings to you, which sums up my 40-plus years of work as a GP and if I were reborn I would still want to be a doctor.

What did you feel when your daughter wanted to become a doctor?

Well, the thing is, her mother, my wife Greta, is a nurse and she used to help me as a practice nurse. When she came to the surgery there were times when she brought Samina with her to help her with bits and pieces. To begin with I did not drive and when I did night visits, Greta had to drive, and Samina had to get up and come with us. Even when she was little she helped, she used to come to the surgery and get the notes out and file them and call the patients in, so that she had that medical feeling from a young age. She learnt a lot from being in the same atmosphere and that is a short cut from the theory of medicine, although that is important too. Samina learnt from being in a home with a medical ambience and seeing me come home in the evening. When I was worried about a patient she would hear me on the phone asking how they were and now I know she does the same thing with her patients as she saw her dad doing. Since those times, general practice has changed beyond recognition.

Quite soon I was able to buy another, larger house and turn that into a surgery and, by 1988, I built a large extension as a treatment room. I have always been an enthusiast of Harold Macmillan, because he was also a humanist; he was a Tory with a passion for human beings so I named my own surgery the Harold Macmillan Medical Centre and I invited his son to be present at the opening ceremony.

When you look back do you think there are any changes for the better in the NHS GP practice?

There are too many managers now in NHS. Managers are supposed to look after the care of the patient in the hospital. Last year my wife had to be admitted to ICU with a heart condition, where the clinical treatment was excellent but there was relatively limited personal care. You often read in the newspapers these days, for example, that the auxiliary staff serve the food, but they put it on the table on one side of the bed and if the patient is too weak to turn over they just come back in an hour and remove it, they do not bother to think. There are too many different languages and cultures being spoken by the auxiliary staff for some of them to understand what the patient needs, or even to care. Tell me, whose responsibility is it when the managers are too busy ticking their boxes? Even worse, elderly patients may be wet with their urine, or toilet, for one week and nobody comes to change their sheets, as reported in the media. Personal care has been relatively neglected, not just in Staffordshire but also all over the UK. If you dare to raise the issue as a doctor your career may be prejudiced for being a whistleblower. My wife received excellent clinical treatment, God saved her and we are grateful for that. What we need now is for patient care to start to be synthesized and the current fragmentation must stop. There is no doubt that medical progress has been made but now significant gaps in care are appearing in our NHS hospitals.

What is the most exciting aspect of developing medical techniques that you have witnessed during your long career?

I think the development of heart techniques is fantastic. Now you can put in a stent, do open-heart surgery, or even a heart transplant, and the progress in kidney surgery is excellent too. The management of diseases like diabetes, hypertension, kidney failure, heart problems and joint replacement is excellent and the treatment options are building up all the time, but the patient care and nursing are not making parallel progress. It is time that the managers were regulated as strictly as the doctors are.

Do you have any observations about cancer?

Cancer is a multi-causation problem. There is a genetic component and if there is a family history of cancer you are more likely to get it. Then there are environmental issues as with bowel cancer whereby the more preservatives and additives we take in our food, the more likely the bowel is to be irritated and become infected. We sometimes misdiagnose, may underdiagnose and, we also over diagnose, as there are some tests that are so sensitive that we are prone to over diagnose and other blood markers are so specific to individual disease that we may miss something else. One always has to draw a balance and consider the history, the clinical findings on examination, and results of various investigations to arrive at a correct diagnosis. I still regard smoking to be the biggest cause of all the problems.

In Pakistan I think I saw more stomach cancer than any other, because of the food and then helicobacter pylori was discovered around 1990. Before that anybody in Pakistan, or here in UK, with an ulcer used to be kept on the ward with a milk drip to soothe the ulcers. If anybody saw a patient having a cigarette on the ward they were immediately asked to go home and told that they couldn't be cured by medicine. But once they discovered helicobacter pylori, which are now known to be 90 per cent of the cause of stomach inflammations and may end up as stomach cancer, the treatment has radically changed. My mother, I think, could not be diagnosed in the 1960s (having helicobacter pylori), ended up with gastric carcinoma, and died of it in 1970. She was only 60 years old when my family rang me from Pakistan and said that Mum was losing weight. They did her barium meal, there was no camera (endoscopy) then, her doctor said it was fine and they sent me the barium-meal films. I showed them to a consultant here and he said, 'This is cancer.' I brought her over but the cancer had spread into her peritoneum. She was operated on but could not be saved. Now, when I look back I think that originally it was an undiagnosed helicobacter infection over the years, which ended up as an inoperable gastric carcinoma.

It is also interesting how prostate cancer has come so much more out in the open because it is more easily diagnosable. When I was a young doctor we only used to see cases of prostate cancer with secondaries when people presented with pain in their hip bone and lower back and a simple X-ray would show the bones were already crushed. Or they might have a severe urinary retention. As a young doctor in Pakistan I used to put my finger into the bladder and pull the prostate out and finish the matter.

Are you saying that in Pakistan you would pull out the prostate without surgery?

Yes, in those days we would put our finger around the prostate and pull it out and that was all. You see, in those days, nobody was so bothered about ejaculation. Prostate makes semen so when you remove the prostate the sex life is destroyed and now people are more thoughtful and demanding and as long as it is an enlargement and without malignancy we can do a different kind of intervention and the management of prostate has become more elaborate and challenging than when we were young doctors. When I was young we were taught that with breast cancer you immediately operated and removed the whole breast and the adjacent muscles as well. A great refinement of surgery has taken place. The treatment becomes superior all the time but the overall management and care of the patients has not made similar progress.

Can you tell me a little about how you have managed the inevitable stresses of being a doctor? You so clearly have not burnt out and your eyes are still full of enthusiasm and a passion for your work.

THE MEANING OF LIFE IS LIFE

My hobbies have been mostly films and books. I was in my fourth year as a medical student when I picked up a book by Aldous Huxley called *Ends and Means* because at that time I wanted to try to understand the meaning of life. I don't know why, but the meaning of life has always been important to me. Then, I picked up another book by Bertrand Russell, *Marriage and Morals* so those two books started me off on my desire to understand the meanings of life. I became interested in films and one of my favourite directors is Ingmar Bergman and his film *Wild Strawberries* and then I read about him in *Time Magazine*, which I read regularly.

Bergman taught me that the meaning of life is 'Life'. You have to live life and that is it. Bergman was my muse and Aldous Huxley gave me mental power. I saw films by Buñuel, who was the partner of Dalí, and they both had the same surreal attitude to life. I also liked very much Fellini and Antonioni. These directors impressed me so much and that gave me another perception on how to live life. Yes, I have found that the meaning of life is life.

Have you continued to have a Muslim faith?

Muslim faith, I have. I learnt another thing from Aldous Huxley. He wrote a book called *The Perennial Philosophy* in which he covered all the religions and found that they all end up in the same way although their journeys and meanings may be very different. I personally feel that our Creator is the same but we all have different roads by which we reach our destination. I have a faith in God, I have a full faith in God, because within borders of our intellect we cannot explain more than that, but by common sense I feel that there has to be somebody who has made all this. Aldous Huxley was also a mystic and believed that we can have ultimate union with God in a trance state.

That is also a Sufi belief.

The Sufis, yes, and each country have their own branch of mysticism. Huxley wrote that the cause and the effect are separate things. How you end up in a certain effect has nothing to do with the journey towards that effect, whether it is to do with being 'bashed up', whipping, hallucinogenic drugs, love, fasting – he insisted that they were separate things. By the way, my name is Mansur and there was a Sufi called Mansur in Baghdad and he said, in Arabic in the trance, 'I am the truth.' People thought that he was claiming to be God and they hanged him. They did not understand his words.

I believe that all the religions have their own route and which one we choose is our personal choice and people should believe whatever they like and I respect everybody's feelings. I know it is not easy to do that but I wish that was the normal thing. The main thing to remember is that there are three aspects of religion: faith, ritual and ethics. Everyone talks about faith and its rituals but the question of ethics is different. Almost everywhere, the people at the forefront of various charities, functions, and celebrations do so with so much enthusiasm and zest that faith is likely to overshadow the aspect of ethics in our day-to-day life.

As a doctor have you found that it is easier for those patients who have faith to accept terminal illness and their death?

Difficult to say, but the third part of every religion is ethics, which is about how we behave with our fellow human beings. Not everybody seems to focus on, or care about, that aspect and yet as a doctor you get a special and extraordinary privilege from God that you can help a fellow human being. What more can anyone ask from life?

THE MEANING OF LIFE IS LIFE

If you had not been a doctor is there any other profession that now appeals to you?

I don't know. Honestly, this is my personal conviction that I am really grateful to God that he made me a doctor, so that I can perform some good to other fellow human beings. Humility and a love for all people are two necessary ingredients of a good doctor. Be a good listener and let the patient talk freely thus guiding the doctor to arrive at his diagnosis. That should be the spirit I think, of every doctor in any country, that you must help any of your fellow human beings who are in pain. I feel humble that I got the chance to help other human beings to the best of my ability. That is what I truly feel.

295

14
MARTIN'S FATHER DIES

All doctors are more than unusually aware of death – though some do their best to hide the metaphysical fact by thinking only in the terms of physiological stages of dying. In the human imagination death and the passing of time are indissolubly linked: each moment that passes brings us nearer to our death and our death if it can be measured at all, is measured by that eternity of existence which must continue after and without us.

John Berger, *A Fortunate Man*

July 2012

In my life thoughts about death are never far away; how can it be different for any dutifully involved general practitioner? We cope – all of us – by reducing our anxiety over the finite nature of our own lives by putting ourselves in a class apart and keeping morbid introspection at arm's length, which works, until we have to confront the loss of a loved one, or if we sustain a potentially lethal illness. I confronted some of these feelings head-on when I calculated, a year or two back, that if I live to be 99, I now have about 200,000 hours left to live: not much.

Yet somehow I still waste my time sitting in traffic on house calls when maybe those patients could come to me. What is that about? Perhaps it is an ingrowing sense of inadequacy in my 'trade', trying to prove something, trying to do something extra. Or perhaps I still value that moment when one enters a patient's home, often at an unseasonable and private hour, presumably to visit someone who is particularly sick and anxious about themselves. Perhaps it is a small child that I have known since birth. With that entrance comes a sense that 'the trusted doctor has arrived'. Meeting one's patients only ever in the context of the consulting room produces a curtailed sense of relationship, reduces the opportunity of indirect 'clues' and emphasizes the 'business'. Or could it be that, in the same way Cosmo has been so influenced by accompanying me on those Saturday morning house visits, they feed into my nostalgia for an unhurried and holistic relationship that has all but disappeared.

Once I left the NHS in 1977 and entered the world of private general practice in the community of West London I realized that care of the dying, in their own homes when possible, was going to be a central activity of my work. I was introduced to this during my time as a GP trainee by my mentor, Dr James Scobie, and it all seemed right, correct, natural and very possible, given the high degree of support that was provided to our dying patients by the practice in which we worked. It was not difficult to translate this training experience into my practice in the independent sector when an immediate need became apparent. Although at the age of 30 I had not had to cope personally with bereavement and loss – with the exception of my four elderly grandparents – I had cared for and been deeply involved with dying patients, both adults and children during my time in the hospital service. Coping with the demands of attending a dying patient at home, their eventual demise, and the subsequent support of the family, was something I could manage and it has continued to be one of the most pivotal and important tasks I have achieved for people under my care.

As I write this I am having the most vivid recollection of the home care of a patient who was 42 and who died at home in Chelsea from colon cancer, the diagnosis having been missed by her previous GP. She was French, with a somewhat older husband who was traditionally English, and they had a daughter aged 11. The woman died early on Christmas morning, when I was with her and her husband then told me that he would take his daughter out for a long walk, if only I could find and arrange for an undertaker to remove his wife's body, all of which I managed to organize. I had to be patient as I drove across Belgrave Square on the way home to my family Christmas much later in the morning as I was stopped and breathalyzed. All through that holiday I could not escape the sense that there was just not enough I could do – my inadequacy surfacing again – for this tragically bereaved man and his daughter and, as I write, that sensation is still alive and uncomfortable as ever. Which leads me to reflect that even though I spend many hours each year in study and research into new medical techniques a doctor never has the luxury of knowing anything for certain. Most of the time you are right and your diagnosis is confirmed by recovery or improvement, or even an inevitable decline. But too often it is a lucky intuition, or unexpected clue, rather than firm knowledge, which leads the race to diagnosis and the inadequacy of my knowledge and the fear of a mistake never completely disappear.

Once I was working in the independent sector a great deal of palliative care came my way. I added to my postgraduate experience with periods of training at St Joseph's Hospice in Hackney and St Columba's Hospice in Edinburgh, which opened the way for me to become the founding Medical Director of a newly opened Palliative Care Unit at the Hospital of St John and St Elizabeth, which is an independent hospital that had remained outside of the NHS when nationalization took place in 1948. The hospital had rather lost its way: run by an ancient Catholic order of nuns, the Order of Mercy, founded in 1218 and which was then under the patronage of the Archbishop of Westminster. The enterprise lacked a modernizing and vigorous approach to healthcare and was slowly becoming a fiefdom for a small number of senior clinicians who enjoyed the old-fashioned and benevolent environment provided by the grand Victorian buildings, the chapel, and its historic and privileged atmosphere. The problem was that without management competence and a profit motive the opportunities for keeping up with the emerging competition – let alone the opportunities for survival – were limited. The hospital was doomed. Then an inspiration came forward to utilize the profits - which could now be made unashamedly – to run a single major charitable endeavor and to open an attached hospice unit, initially styled as the Catherine McAuley Unit, and subsequently St John's Hospice was born. We had a humble beginning with just five beds, but grew over a few years to 18 beds and more, with a vibrant day-care scheme and the important commitment, through attached Macmillan nurses, to home care. I held the post for some years until eventually we were in the position to replace me with a full-time Consultant in Palliative Care, and an expanding professional team.

Over a period of more than three decades there have been many patients who have died under my care and of course every experience has been different, though each death is equally arduous, and only made possible by a self imposed contract of continuity of care and the commitment to being present, which is only possible by making constant availability the watchword. When somebody is dying the terrors that may accompany their journey can at least be mitigated by the doctor's, or his deputy's 'promise', to visit the home and family at almost any time of day and night. As I write this I realize that it sounds like an anachronism but less than 20 years ago it was what was expected of any family doctor and his team.

As the years have passed I cannot forget any one of those experiences for they continue to dominate my memory. As I pass the homes of the deceased, meet their relatives on other occasions, I feel in touch with and reminded of those people. Apart from the home care I have provided to such patients at the end of serious illness there are also those people who have died suddenly and unexpectedly in accidents, or as a result of acute and brief illness. How will I ever forget the mother of three children, aged 30, who died of influenza after calling our surgery at 9 am to request a home visit. She was seen at midday but by then she was already so ill that even though I immediately called an ambulance by the time we reached hospital she was so overwhelmed with viraemia (blood poisoning) that she died four hours later. Or, the two brothers who died in a light aircraft in the Alps; our pathology technician who died in a fall from her horse; the banker who fell asleep in his car on the motorway when driving to his country house late on a Friday night at the end of a heavy week. These descriptions are but a minuscule few of the remembered dead and every one and many more return to my mind; some of them almost daily. Their names are etched on to the stubs of what reminds me of a chequebook that will never run dry but which in reality is my book of certificates stating the Cause of Death. Yes, the truncation of death fixes itself into my memory with indelible ink.

After a while in practice I realized that one of the most important but ill-recognized qualifications for a GP such as myself was parenthood. I was 34 when my first child, Cosmo, was born and that birth is a moment that has remained transcendent. I delivered Cosmo in Guy's Hospital myself. His mother was exhausted, as she had only been discharged from the hospital on the previous day. She had contracted pneumonia late in her pregnancy while living on the Paediatric ward at the hospital following the diagnosis of acute juvenile diabetes in Ben, her first son, who was then aged seven. I quickly found myself juggling several balls: on call for the weekend (it was a Saturday night), new baby, wife with hypertension, renal failure, recent pneumonia, and a stepson with acute diabetes on four injections of insulin daily. It was a normal weekend for a multitasking GP.

I wrapped up our baby in a warm towel; he gave a tiny cry, no it was more of a murmur, a predictor of his future self. Cosmo rarely complains and he never shouts loud as he has never been one to make a fuss. I carried him to the window, ever aware of the need to manage the third stage of labour and to deliver the placenta but there was just a moment for me to show him to the world, from the fourteenth floor, with HMS Belfast moored in the Thames far below. I am told that in your lifetime your heart does enough work to lift that great battleship 18 inches out of the water, and I told this to Cosmo. He looked like a little purple frog, and I thought, quite unexpectedly and involuntarily, about my own eventual death, and the fact that my swaddled son would no doubt be there, looking after me in my demise as I was now looking after him, at his birth. Just for a second I was moved, so slightly, until that sense of inadequacy reared its presence for another moment. How could I possibly be any good as a parent?

My father died on 6 July 2012 after being ill for several days. He was 92 and when he died he had been demented for more than four years. I remember how, 10 years ago, he said, 'Don't give me any more books, don't give me a book for Christmas! I can't follow them any more.' I thought, 'Here we go,' and knew then he was developing dementia.

Did he know?

I think he did, because he admitted that reading was becoming too difficult and he had occasional falls, and then he broke his finger and couldn't hold his walking stick. He became more and more obsessive and started to lose track of time – he became very difficult to manage.

Now you are 62 does it create anxiety thinking about your father?

Well, the one anxiety it has created for the last five years is that I have been fearing that my big enemy is going to be dementia and I suppose it's also because I'm at the age where I can see myself losing aspects of my memory; I have become particularly bad with names. I console myself by telling anxious patients, 'If your memory was once really, really good you notice it when it starts to fragment a bit, whereas if your memory was never any good it wouldn't make that much difference.' When I was younger – if I met you in the supermarket – I would not only know your name and mobile number but also your car-registration plate. My father had a Morris 1100: OLT 300E. I am becoming hopeless at names, and while I'm aware that that is not dementia it still makes me anxious. What, with my father living into his nineties, and how I want to remain independent, healthy and active until I am a hundred. Now I worry that I could develop a dementia like him but then he was a very, very heavy drinker, which I am not and I'm very active which he was not. His entry in *Who's Who* included gardening but that involved putting the window up and telling the gardener what to do.

Was he forced to retire at 65?

No, well, yes from the NHS but then he carried on as a private anaesthetist until he was 70 and he was still politically involved with various committees and the final edition of his book. No, I am not like him but then maybe there's more to getting Alzheimer's, or the sort of dementia he had.

You never wanted to diagnose it.

Mother wouldn't have allowed it and what's the point. In fact, you cannot get an accurate diagnosis of dementia without a brain biopsy, which nobody does, or there are some very fancy modern sorts of scans but which are only of research value.

When did he die? Were you there?

No. In fact, he had quite a journey that week. On the Monday, Mother called the GP in the morning but a nurse came. Then my mother thought she was calling in the GP but she had called an ambulance. Barnet General Hospital, on arrival, said, 'We don't do urology.' The ambulance took Father on to Chase Farm Hospital but they couldn't admit him because the lifts were out of order. He spent three hours in the ambulance and eventually was admitted and then sent home after his catheter was changed. He became difficult, even aggressive and then spent the day hollering. My brother agreed with me that he had to be allowed to go without any more medication but then he stopped eating and drinking and – by the way – his NHS GP for many years never visited him once. Mother rang me and said, 'He's just spoken, he said clearly: "I am broken."' He became comatose and I tried to explain to Mother that he was going to die. The next morning she went down at about 5.20 am and found him dead in his bed. Mother phoned me and said, 'Your father's stopped breathing.' I thought, 'Thank God for that.' We got the undertakers, Clark's of

Barnet, and that is important because Tony Clark was my parents' best man and Bob Clark, who was Tony's brother, was the first GP who trained me in general practice. Interestingly, Bob and Tony Clark died within an hour of each other. One was on a plane and the other was conducting a GP surgery and they both died in the same hour from coronaries. The undertaker asked what coffin we wanted and I replied that we wanted the cheapest, which they said was, '£80 but we do a good oak for £800.' He would have hated that expenditure, so I said, 'Chipboard it will be.' Father always believed that he didn't have any money and he was parsimonious in spirit as well. One of his favourite phrases was, "Do not dilute the argument. That is irrelevant." He was an aggressive father, but he was a great committee man because he wouldn't tolerate any diversions. He never did 'chit-chat', and even in his obituary it was noted that his colleagues had often referred to him as 'laconic, shy and taciturn'.

I noticed in his obituary that he was also one of the first clinicians to bring up issues about professional fitness to practise.

Yes, but that was ironical, because everybody knew that he would go to the hospital bar at lunch time and then straight on to the ward to anaesthetize a patient but they all did, it was de rigueur. He was part of the 'Gin and Jaguar' set of consultants, except he had no interest in cars.

Do you have any regrets when you think about him?

I have so many regrets but who wouldn't? I've ended up knowing so little about him. I tried so hard with him but he was always inaccessible. Even his obit in the BMJ commented on how silent he was. When his mother had dementia he once – uncharacteristically intimate – said to me, 'Do you know I said goodbye to my mother years ago.' Years later I would think to myself, 'I don't need to say goodbye to you, because you haven't said "Hello" yet.' I never felt that he said 'Hello' to me. As I said I went to the funeral, I did everything necessary, but I've never cried, in fact the nearest I have got to feeling teary was speaking to you just now, when I mentioned the time of his death. Now it feels sad but both my brother and me were business-like about his death, that is how we function together, distanced. We are a distant family. Anyway, my script is that it was time for him to go. The family all went to the funeral and I also had three ex's there.

What was the day of the funeral?

Well, it must have been 20 July. I could look in my diary. It was raining. We came out of the church and it was pissing with rain. My mother sent everyone to the church hall but I said, 'No I am coming to the grave,' where there was all this false grass laid out and the lovely vicar, in a huge brimmed hat, said some prayer type stuff and offered around a tray with some earth on it and two of us stepped forward. I thought, 'Well, he is in the ground, which is what he wanted and I've chucked some soil on him,' and that was that. I haven't been back to the grave. I probably won't reach my father's age and he was still so frightened of dying. He was so frightened, but then he was frightened of everything, being cut open, or anaesthetized. I always think, 'God, how unsympathetic must you have been as a clinician.' For him, medicine was always only a practical physiology experiment.

He was disappointed that he didn't end up with a knighthood and only a CBE. That is what happens to anaesthetists; they end up being regarded as very posh nurses but they are the really

305

clever ones, not the surgeons. It is the most finely tuned skill of all, as Cosmo has already told you. Yes, my father was absolutely brilliant with his hands and he wouldn't do anything practical with them, not like me, I've wrecked my hands doing things.

Your account of your organizational skills when he died sounds as though you followed immaculate protocol and gave him every respect that his life deserved but I still have no idea what you felt. Did it release any feelings, emotions, knowing that he was gone forever?

I am a bit torn here between the act that I put on and the feelings that I have because I sort of live in the act. I say to people – I'm not sure if I'm still believing the script – because I say to people, 'I'm glad he died. He needed to go,' and I think for a long while I just kept wishing he would die. I knew my mother needed to be released from the absolute and eternal purgatory of nursing him. In fact she is doing magnificently and you know I have never been a great admirer of hers for lots of reasons. Her care was absolute. He died weighing about six stone but without a bedsore, lovingly cared for at home, and in the end he had to be confined to his bed because he was always trying to escape. He had cot sides, which you are not allowed any more in the NHS but it stopped him from falling out.

Have you ever thought about what sort of father you would have liked?

Yes, insofar as with my own children I've tried to be the sort of father I didn't get. But now it's a more liberal society and I've changed my babies' nappies and taken care of the kids. I've tried

MARTIN'S FATHER DIES

to teach my children practical skills like using a drill, or being interested in their projects, 'This is how you do it, that is how you use a hammer, help me to put the decking down, we'll do it together.' I'd also like to think I've talked a bit to them about the things he didn't. He never once spoke to me about women. Everything was about him being critical of my failures, not getting into Cambridge, not getting three As at A-level, I just felt endlessly criticized. It has made me endlessly aim for betterment and turned me into being a people pleaser. I think those reflexes become innate. You spend your time trying to do good work and to be punctual and I was so minimally rebellious. When I see rebellion now, I think, 'Good on you.' You know young people come in covered in tattoos and piercings and I wonder whether their parents roll their eyes but I was just obedient. The most outrageous thing I ever did was to say, 'I'm going to the Windsor Jazz Festival,' which was immediately opposed with negative propositions by my father. Now, I can remember coming home one evening, not late, I was a medical student and my mother was sitting on the stairs waiting for me and she said, 'I am sick of your affairs with older women.' Probably it was alcohol speaking, but she was obviously terribly jealous of the permissive generation with the pill. I don't think she had a wildly fun time with my father. He might have been sexually demanding but there was no night-clubbing.

Your father has moulded you by default.

Yes, and I have tried to redress it with my sons and to give them enough money but not too much, plenty but not too much, but I do want to indulge them. I have given them both cars and seen they have had all the things you need to take girls out and to have an independent adult life while they are students. I

307

hope I've given them enough wherewithal. Perhaps I have been financially better off than he was, and I've forgiven him now, but he was very mean. Yes, he was blooming mean, and from the minute I qualified and we went out as a family I paid; I paid for everything. If I go out with Cosmo now, I pay – he at 28 is not paying for me.

If it were Cosmo sitting here reminiscing about your life, would you hope for memories of more emotional engagement?

Well, that is an interesting question. I wouldn't want him to be crying, or terribly distraught about my death, not so that he couldn't go to work.

Don't you think there is something valuable about grieving? As you know I didn't grieve for my mother either but I regret that. I regret that I didn't grieve for my mother. It is a great loss not to miss a parent.

I'm sure, if I died tonight, Cosmo would be distraught because he is more emotional than me, although he doesn't show it to me. He probably knows that he shouldn't, because I must have signalled to him through my body language that he's not to. He came to the practice last week with tonsillitis, not to get treatment, but to collect some medicines from our pharmacy for his emergency kit. I said, 'Are you not very well?' and he said, 'Not really, I've got tonsillitis again.' 'Are you taking something?' and he replied, 'I've put myself on something.' We were in the pharmacy and Chris the pharmacist was there, and I thought to myself, 'I'd like to give you a hug Cosmo, but we don't do that, we don't do giving each other a hug, Cosmo and I.' We have fallen out of the habit, if it ever existed. I might squeeze his arm but that's as far as it gets. I felt my love but we don't enact it.

Cosmo will read in our transcript that his dad thought he wanted to give his son a hug. Sad and beautiful.

Yes, but then he is standing there, two inches taller than me with whiskers on his chin, he is a great hunky bloke.

Who, Cosmo? He doesn't look like 'a great hunky bloke', even if he is taller than you. Cosmo is slight, like you were. If I think of my son, Alex and his father dying, I think he would be devastated. They often row in the kitchen when they cook together, as Alex is like a health-and-safety official when they are cooking. He loves to criticize his father, but he adores him. I think Alex might be stunned for days.

Well, I think Cosmo and Mylo, my other son, who decided not to go into medicine but strategy at PriceWaterhouse PLC would be too if I died, but I think Cosmo would go straight back to work because that is what would make him feel better. If I died I would want Cosmo to feel, 'Well, Dad had a jolly good life, he loved everything, he was passionate about medicine to the end, he was surrounded by women, fabulous birds, he loved cars, he had loads of them, he always wanted a tractor and he got one, he got everything he wanted so Amen to that, even if he was run over at 62.' I never saw my father rejoice in anything, let alone anything that I have achieved. I think he had just about enough wit left to see my newspaper column, to see my picture, so I hope he might have been a bit proud of that even though it was the *Daily Mail*.

15

OH! THERE IS SO MUCH I COULD SPEAK ABOUT DEATH

Natasha's journey towards medicine as a mature student has been one in which she has acquired many degrees on her way, both academic and in the school of life, which will be discovered in the course of her narrative She is currently working as a Junior Doctor in Bristol while she makes the decision whether, postgraduation, to train as a GP or psychiatrist.

Natasha and I – strangers minutes before – found ourselves beginning our meeting by talking about orifices. Natasha got in touch with me after Gwen, one of her closest friends, had sent her our interview to censor, or approve. Natasha then expressed interest in coming up from Bristol for her own interview. I had not yet started recording as Natasha described how doctors have an incredibly privileged access to our bodies, which she referred to as the 'legitimized breach of bodily boundaries', and how acts that doctors undertook on a daily basis which breach boundaries (surgery, rectal and vaginal examinations, inserting urinary catheters, etc.) can become routine for them while remaining sensitive for patients. Also, that the gender and power issues these acts entail are little discussed at medical school.

I don't entirely understand the British squeamishness about the anus. It's interesting because my last job as a junior doctor before my current paediatric rota was in colorectal surgery, a challenging job because there were people on the ward who were my age with colorectal cancer, which was harrowing at times. My clinical experience has made me reflect on British cultural politics around the anus, especially as I grew up in France where suppositories were a routine way for children to be given medicines. There is almost a rule in paediatrics in the UK that you don't go near a child's bottom, you can have a look but you only carry out an examination if it is critical, and suppositories are only prescribed for emergencies. On the colorectal and care of the elderly wards you are often doing rectal examinations every day, but with children it's quite different. We were taught at medical school that 'If you don't put your finger in it, you will put your foot in it', but I would never do an anal examination with children as a junior doctor. With adults I always try to remember that even if I'm doing examinations five times a day, they can still be experienced as very intrusive. I think busy, stressed doctors can forget that there is a personal history attached to bodily parts. I had a patient last year who was very young - in his early twenties, street-savvy, tough-looking - who desperately needed a urinary catheter because he was in urinary retention post-operatively (which is agony), but who became very distressed when he was advised he had to have one. I talked to him and he was weeping, refusing outright and begging for alternatives. I slowly realized that he was signaling to me indirectly that he had been abused horribly as a child. My senior surgical colleagues refused to listen and told me to tell him that he HAD to have one otherwise he risked bladder perforation, when the compassionate approach could have been to consider a supra-pubic catheter (which did not involve his penis). The situation appalled me.

Martin speaks elsewhere in the book about how fazed he was as a boy when the GP just turned him over and anally examined

him. I had a similar experience when I was about ten and had a suspected appendicitis. I felt both humiliated and ashamed but also vaguely excited, particularly as the surgeon was the most handsome man I had ever seen.

I have done many rectal examinations, as well as watching them being done during my training, and they have generally been carried out sensitively and with an explanation of the procedure. I think that life-experience is crucial to becoming a sympathetic doctor and to knowing that to become a patient is to fall into one of the most vulnerable states there is. My first non-professional experience of being in hospital was when my newborn baby son, Isaac, was the patient. It was six years ago and happened after a normal delivery, after which I didn't leave Intensive Care at all for a month. I couldn't drag myself away from Isaac for even one minute. I was already at medical school but I hadn't done any clinical training and I didn't feel medically knowledgeable in any useful way. I didn't know what was wrong with my son and nobody else did either. It was a humbling experience for me. We were stranded in the Intensive Care Unit, and in effect I became an ethnographer as I spent 18 hours a day watching what was taking place around me. There were some wonderful nurses and we talked, but I didn't have a normal postnatal period at all, although I was able to spend a lot of time skin to skin and just holding Isaac kangaroo-close. I was in a very sensory environment and being bombarded with sound. It was a shocking time, watching babies born around 23 weeks struggle for life. I always thought Isaac was on the wrong ward because he was nearly nine pounds when he came out and it was a normal delivery. Giving birth to my son was a triumphal experience but even that intensity of emotion could not be compared to the intensity of pain of losing my loved ones, of seeing somebody you love slip away in front of your eyes.

OH! THERE IS SO MUCH I COULD SPEAK ABOUT DEATH

Intensive Care was like being in a parallel universe. If you give birth to a baby you think you've made it, you have managed not to have a premature delivery (probably my greatest fear), and you have got through all the drama of birth. I managed a natural vaginal one, and then you think you are on firm ground. In fact, Isaac's illness was the start of a slippery journey for me towards thinking that medicine is not what it makes itself out to be quite a lot of the time. I am very aware of the power that medical culture asserts in all domains and it's easy to get seduced by that power as a medic because it is a position of enormous privilege, enormous privilege. I am not sure that this is always sufficiently in people's consciousness when they do medicine, particularly if they haven't also personally experienced a contrasting position of vulnerability. I don't think medicine is good at embracing uncertainty and that is why both general practice and psychiatry appeal to me. Both necessarily embrace this uncertainty while everything else is moving towards evidence-based medicine. Even general practice is moving in that direction, despite the possibility that in doing so, important other qualities like intuition, doubt, even uncertainty and patience are sacrificed.

Yes, and perhaps it is no surprise that it was John Keats, who was studying medicine before he became a poet, and who later as a poet coined the invaluable phrase in a letter to his brother, of 'Negative Capability', by which he meant attaining a state of mind where one could endure uncertainty without becoming 'irritable' and driven to find 'truth'.

Isaac's medical story was a surprising one and full of uncertainty. He presented with low blood sugar, not an uncommon symptom in the newborn, but the situation deteriorated very rapidly and he was found to be profoundly hypoglycaemic. I was both a mother

313

of a newborn and a medical student who didn't yet suffer from knowing too much. That is the doctor's burden when we become a parent, or someone we love falls ill.

As a doctor one is taught that common things are common and you must think of them first, which means that serious things are sometimes missed even though they are right under your nose. In Isaac's case none of the doctors had any idea what was wrong with him as he had no clinical signs and presented as normal. The blood tests got more and more obscure and took longer and longer to come back. It was only when the neonatal doctors started talking to the endocrine team at the children's hospital, who had requested specific blood tests relating to the pituitary gland that it came to light that he was congenitally deficient in several pituitary hormones. We now know that Isaac has a condition that is one or two in a million, and it fascinates me that we all take our pituitary glands for granted.

I am not even sure where mine is. Somewhere in my head, I think.

It really intrigues me that people know about the pancreas and insulin but the pituitary gland, which is actually the size of a pea, is culturally invisible. When surgeons want to get to it to remove a tumour, it is reached through your nose. It's attached to part of the neural tissue of the hypothalamus and is involved in a complex messaging network for the whole body and without which we would not survive, or be walking around. It signals to the adrenal glands to make cortisol, which keeps us alive when we are extremely unwell or biologically stressed, and also triggers the production of reproductive, thyroid and growth hormones. It is the master gland of our bodies and Galen, the ancient medic, first wrote about it in 150 AD. (He thought its purpose was to drain phlegm from the brain.) I think in Eastern traditions, which conceptualize our bodies very differently, it is connected to the third eye.

This was all happening to you after losing your mother two years earlier?

I remember when we were able to leave the hospital and I put Isaac into his car seat, it felt like we had come to the end (or beginning) of a journey. I sat in the back with Isaac and cried all the way home. My only thought was, 'I don't have a mother any more, my mother has gone.'

Perhaps we should go back to the beginning. I know that you were a distinguished medical anthropologist before you decided to train to be a doctor. Is that what you read at Cambridge?

No, I read Classics at Cambridge. I have a very long story and my earliest interests were the literary arts and music.

Oh, you are a modest polymath.

Well, I don't seem able to stop learning. And now I am combining being a junior doctor in A&E along with doing molecular biology. I'm also an academic doctor who is still trying to decide whether to specialize as a GP, or a psychiatrist.

DOCTORS DISSECTED

Tell me a little about your family.

I had a happy childhood and felt unconditionally loved, and I think you can divide the world into those who have and have not been. My mother was a teacher and I was close to her. I was the last born of four. I loved school and was brilliant at it and then I followed my heart to do an Arts degree.

You haven't mentioned your father...

My father [LONG PAUSE] has always been supportive and still lives in London. He worked in administration. He speaks of himself as an under-achiever and both of my parents were the first members of their families to get a degree. They both came from the North. There are parts of my family history that remain a little bit murky and there are all sorts of skeletons in the cupboard, but my understanding is that my parents left England for a new start in France in the mid 1960s, where they stayed for the next 20 years. I often felt as the youngest child that I was looking in from the outside of the family matrix and not quite understanding what I saw. My father suffered from migraines and 'the black dog', and in fact I am convinced that every member of my immediate family has suffered from undiagnosed depression. My father's mother had electroshock therapy in the 1950s but I don't have any details.

I am the only child to get a degree in the family, and I have four degrees as my brother Tom jokes, one for each of them. Early on, as far back as I can remember, being good at what I did brought me recognition and I became an overachiever, something I still struggle to contain. I remember at the age of five going to Knossos in Crete and sitting on the Minoan throne. I was passionately interested in Greek myth as a child, and I still have all my childhood editions to show my son at some point. I was a pretty intense teenager and I was also passionate about music and studied it at A-level. Playing in the Youth Orchestra was one highlight of my life. Yes, I am goal orientated, but that has helped me through medical school where you always have to jump hurdles.

I loved Cambridge where I had an archetypal Arts student experience. I listened to Bob Dylan endlessly, smoked ganja and drank with the arts crowd. I also had a passionate love affair, which lasted for several years. In my third year at Cambridge I did a module with Germaine Greer called Ancient Erotics, which led me to feminist theory, gender issues and narratives of the body. I went to one of Germaine's afternoon parties where she revelled in the attention of beautiful young things.

I have also always been interested in Africa; I can't explain that, it just is. In the mid 1980s when the South African townships were burning and there were all those horrific massacres, I watched it all happening as a teenager on TV and I remember thinking, 'What must it be like to live there and be in the middle of all that?' I had never heard of Medical Anthropology and was considering Medicine after Cambridge but I couldn't imagine going straight into another degree and wanted to travel. Yet, I ended up at the School of African and Oriental Studies in London doing an MA in Medical Anthropology. I finished my Masters when I was 21 and thought the world was my oyster. I left my boyfriend and went off to West Africa with a one-way ticket and various contacts from the university. I ended up in Cape Town working for the Medical Research Council, which led me to be away for five years and to do a Ph.D on the Anthropology of Violence and Sexual Health. It was 1995, just a year after the first South African elections and it was thrilling. I felt very secure as my early attachments to my parents had been so firm that I felt able to take physical risks and go 'native' in a township.

Having talked to you on the phone I know there is also a tragic element because when you did come back from South Africa you found your mother to be ill with as yet undiagnosed cancer.

Yes. Exactly. [LONG PAUSE]

How were you perceived in the townships?

Well, the fact that I was British and not a white local, helped me because Britain was associated with the anti apartheid struggle. I never saw another white person in the township except the visitors that I took there. I worked with a particular young man who was unemployed but became my link to the township community. I was doing participant observation, like Malinowski and Mead, and writing a field diary. I wanted to understand how the people constructed their story about suffering from HIV, because the doctors wouldn't admit them to hospital as there was simply nothing that could be done for them. Antivirals were not yet available to the Third World. What struck me most was that so many of those young people, stricken by financial poverty and poverty of opportunity, felt out of control of their lives and their sexuality. I was interested in why people used condoms, or decided not to and how this fitted with the micro politics of multiple sexual partnerships. The local language was Xhosa, which is Mandela's language. Most also spoke some English and ghetto slang, the slang of criminal lifestyles, so it was a complex linguistic soup. I heard a lot of things that are usually not accessible to a woman, like narratives about group rape and things like that. I would say 'gang', not 'group' rape, which is what it amounted to, but that word carries so many media connotations, which are confusing. Perhaps most heartbreaking of all was the poverty. You have to live in the midst of poverty to realize its power to drag people down and to make them hopeless, to see the way it steals away all opportunity of equality.

Did you fall in love?

I did have an African boyfriend but he was not part of the township. I was somewhat fought over in all sorts of ways. I had two relationships with African men, both complicated. Being a young white woman with fair hair meant that there was a lot of sexual competition over me. It was complicated with the women too and I really had to work at those relationships. It was also critical that I learnt to read body language to be able to intuit danger, or affection. In many ways I was living in a war zone and half of the young people I worked with are now dead, either from HIV or from violence. Reading body language has remained an important skill for me as a doctor and I am hypersensitive to the patients' unspoken language now when I am on ward rounds.

It was a critical time in the HIV epidemic, because many of the people had been asymptomatically ill for nearly a decade and young people in their twenties were just becoming visibly sick. When I was there, a quarter of pregnant women tested positive for HIV and literally every family was affected in one way or another. As I said, there was nothing at all that could be done and it was devastating to see young people dying in hordes and the elders wringing their hands in hopelessness. I was so involved with one young man that when he died the family asked me to do the 'cause of death' speech at his funeral. This is a traditional ritual, which also happened in communities in the UK a hundred years ago. I had to use language especially sensitively on that day.

DOCTORS DISSECTED

I have had experience of clients who found themselves in a state of melancholia from which they could not recover, as opposed to grief, after somebody they loved has died. They had been excluded from any detailed information about the death, and had not been able to see the body. We no longer have any education in death and the dying, except perhaps in hospices.

It was the community's right to know how the person died. It is so important that these things are named. Death needs to be named. There is something very deep in human nature that does not want to confront death. Doctors may not consciously want to think about it, but they all have to walk in the valley of the shadow of death. Later on, I went to a world AIDS conference in Toronto where I named all the dead from the township as part of an art installation.

'Let me remember you one by one. L – you were the first. I sat by your bedside, minute after long minute, hour after long hour. As you faded away bit by bit, you lost your voice - you literally stopped speaking. Your eyes expressed the anguish of your suffering. Later, I filed past your dead body with the others as the lamenting screamed in the background. You no longer looked like you because too much time had passed. I was there on the bright breezy day when you were buried on a hillside in your ancestral village and when the preacher talked of things being upside down. The women sang and danced for joy, and the cowbells rang out. For them, you had gone to a parallel universe, a better one.'

Most, but not all of the doctors that I have talked to don't want to go into the specifics of death but rather shrug it off as something almost routine, which of course it has to become, but...

Very young doctors have to certify death, that is often the job of the junior doctors, and many of them will not have seen death before. My experience in South Africa was unusual because I saw people after they had died in the heat and before they were buried. Wasted bodies on young people are quite shocking things to see, but I knew that I wanted to be – I don't know how to explain it – I wanted to be close to those huge moments of energy and release.

It fascinates me how you left the ivory towers of Classics to enter what must have felt like the underworld. You wanted to witness the disfigurement of disease and poverty and maybe to offer up some small acts of consolation.

It's famous in Medicine if you want to see pathology you go to Africa and I don't like the way it can become a voyeuristic thing in lectures, 'Look at this wasted African body…look at this clinical sign.' There is nothing that can shock me about the human body any more although every death is shocking. What was particularly awful was that I knew these wasted bodies had suffered often without even the smallest relief granted by paracetamol. I lost my innocence in Africa.

I suddenly have to tell you that, although I have been suffering from depression since the beginning of the year, since my nephew died, that when I was on the train today coming up to London to meet you, the sun began to shine across the countryside. I was listening to opera arias and watching the light and I suddenly thought how much I loved the English countryside; my mood momentarily became ecstatic.

We stopped our first interview here and agreed to meet again the following week.

321

Yes, my family was hugely relieved to have me home after five years in South Africa, although I then became a virtual recluse for a year while I wrote up my thesis. I came back to find my friends were settling down – I was 29 and they were having white weddings and talking about which sofa to buy – I was burned out by the suffering I had witnessed and found it alienating. My mother played an important role in beginning to process my experience because she was a good listener, but she also seemed tired. I had a waking dream like a vision when I came back of my mother dying, which was a year before she was diagnosed with cancer. The week I was about to fly back to South Africa, we were having a family lunch and my mother disappeared into the toilet for a very long time. I thought she had diarrhoea but in truth she was haemorrhaging. That week she was diagnosed with a cancerous tumour of the cervix. She already had a slight cough, which she described as just a little tickle but later on we discovered that she had secondaries in her lungs. She had turned a blind eye to all the early symptoms. Her denial was monumental. For my whole life I remembered a poster in her room of a climber climbing up a vertical cliff and just before she died she confided to me that that was what her life had felt like. I understood then that she had been depressed but unable to face it. It was a kind of suicide. That enabled me to be more forgiving of her than some of my siblings, whom I suspected of judging her for not getting help earlier.

How old was your mother?

I think she was 65 when she was diagnosed, and she wouldn't even tell my father to begin with, so I became her advocate, both in the family and then in the hospital.

OH! THERE IS SO MUCH I COULD SPEAK ABOUT DEATH

Suddenly you were engaged in your mother's dying body, so did that tip returning to South Africa out of your mind?

Yes, I flew back to South Africa for 24 hours to explain to my boss, who was also my good friend, that I wasn't going to take up the job that I had by then been offered. She couldn't believe it and was very unsupportive about the fact that I could sacrifice my international anthropological career to looking after my mother.

Was that from a sense of love or duty?

I think it was love. I felt that my mother nurtured me enormously as a child. It wasn't duty; I wanted to be with her and to give back some of what she had done for me. She had become very vulnerable.

You weren't then a medical doctor but did you immediately see the significance of her symptoms?

I don't think I had got there by then, but she had looked unwell for so many months. She put it down to stress at work and I had watched her breathless and struggling to play tennis. In a complicated way, there was almost a relief in knowing the truth. As I said I had an extraordinary dream soon after her diagnosis that illustrates this. I am in an airport and get detained on my journey by the lack of a boarding card. A man takes me into a room. He has something to show me. The room is empty except for a glass box covered in a cloth. Inside there is an eagle, upright and still, as if stuffed, but I understand that it is not dead. As I watch, the colour in the box reddens and spreads, I don't understand at first then see it is blood threatening to engulf the eagle. At first I am frightened, then as I stand there I see the eagle is beginning to rise up out of the blood. When I wake up, I think, 'Phoenix rising from the ashes,' and I know it is me.

Now, I would put two and two together, at least I think so, but there is a bit of a history in our family of not being able to see what's under our noses, especially if the deterioration is gradual. My nephew, who died a year ago at the age of 12, was quite breathless for several months.

Was that your brother's or sister's child? Was he misdiagnosed with asthma?

My next brother's son, the one I am very close to. Billy was his only child. Before he died last December (2012), he had already had an emergency admission to hospital three years before. The doctors missed the fact that his ECG was abnormal and they didn't do a scan of his heart, which is what he needed. My medical training came too late to help him by a few years, which saddens me enormously, but the GPs and paediatricians missed the diagnosis. He had an aggressively rare lung disease, which is notorious for being the master of disguise. With Billy I didn't feel like a medic at all when it was happening although I had qualified six months previously, because the emotional devastation was overwhelming. Billy was like my own child, a big brother to my son, Isaac. With both Billy and my mother's death, what I still carry with me is the extraordinary defences that people can put up even though their bodies are disintegrating. I found my mother's doctors and oncologists at Guy's Hospital were very sensitive to the fact that she didn't want to know the true prognosis and they didn't push it. My mother never addressed her dying.

OH! THERE IS SO MUCH I COULD SPEAK ABOUT DEATH

Did you want to know?

I knew that it was bad from the moment that she was diagnosed because I had noticed that she had this little dry cough. Her doctors were brilliant at maintaining a sense of hope; they were not lying to her but they were sensitive to her denial and the fact that she didn't want to discuss her prognosis.

It's interesting that she had a little dry cough, and although I am not a doctor I know that an innocuous dry cough that doesn't go away is an example of 'Things greater are in less contain'd'. I seem to know both too little and too much and sometimes I wish I were like my husband who knows nothing about medicine and thinks everything is innocuous until forced to see otherwise. Whenever I have a client with an obstinate dry cough, let alone breathlessness, I insist they see their GP. I've also seen someone die of acute leukaemia who to begin with had nothing more than an innocent cough that wouldn't go away.

Yes…yes and this is something I had not understood before. I've now learnt, having practised as a medic for just over a year, that signs of illness can be very, very subtle and then quick to escalate. People have very different experiences of cancer but my mother had three years of suffering. Her illness taught me that people's relationships with their bodies are highly complex, in that they are a function of personal histories. Doctors can forget that very easily and be frustrated that patients did not seek help earlier. And yet there are all kinds of historical and subconscious influences at work in a person's response to their body. Hospital doctors work with bodies (and body parts if they are surgeons) but I think the complexity of someone's relationship with their symptoms and disintegrating body can be profound, and it is not

325

something that is addressed at medical school where it's often about understanding the physiology. GPs are often the most aware of this complexity because they have to work with it.

My mother died at home, partly because I enabled it and she wanted to die at home because of the privacy. A month before she died I went back to South Africa to complete a project and because one of the young men I was working with was dying of AIDS. I didn't realize then that my mother was on death's doorstep, quite literally.

Was that an instance of denial?

No. She had been fading away for so long that I stopped seeing the gradual decline in front of my eyes. That is what happened with Billy's breathlessness as well. It was a profoundly moving trip for me in every way because the dying young man that I have spoken of was surprised to find me beside his bed. He looked up and into my eyes and said, 'Natasha, I just wish you could be my doctor.' Poignantly he was an HIV educator who was unable to face up to his own illness and diagnosis and he died at 26 because he started antiretrovirals too late.

Was his response to you another factor in your deciding to become a doctor?

Fairly soon after my mother was diagnosed I decided that the only thing I now wanted to do with my life was to become a doctor. I would spend hours lying awake and trying to work out how I could do that as an Arts graduate with no A-level Sciences. I was 30 and I knew I had to do it then or to spend the rest of my life regretting it. I found out six weeks before my mother died that I had been accepted to study Medicine at Bristol, where they were offering me a year's pre-med to catch up on the sciences. My mentors in Anthropology were taken aback that I was about to abandon such a successful and published career. It wasn't that I ascribed any great healing powers to becoming a doctor, but rather that I feel most myself when I am working with people who are very distressed or vulnerable. Being a doctor provides a very privileged way into suffering.

I feel that too, and I have to question myself as to why it should be so.

Yes, I have often wondered about it. I was questioning myself on the train coming to see you today, why is that so? I was nurtured as a child and didn't experience early trauma.

Yes, the greatest emotional challenges have come to you as an adult, whereas my trauma has been generally spread across my life but somehow there is for me the sense of making myself whole through a constant immersion in suffering and reparation.

I feel like I am fulfilling myself, that all of myself, my life journey, is being used in my encounters with patients. I have always had the sense in my family of there being secrets, of my mother holding the whole act together, and then when she was dying it felt like I was taking over her role. I have always been a very responsible person who follows things through and I am loyal. I understand it better now, my wanting to be with people in distress and working with them. My mother knew before she died that I had been accepted at medical school and she also knew my long term partner, so she had a sense of what my life was to become, which does comfort me.

How did you cope with her body and its demise?

My mother was fortunate because she didn't have much pain, but she found the exhaustion very difficult and in the last few days I used to wash her feet. Anointing her feet was the most comforting thing I could do for her. She wanted to have her hair washed the day before she died. She thought it was too difficult but I insisted.

I remember thinking, in my mother's last few days, that if I sat next to her on the sofa she became very hot. She wanted to be in her own space, as she was when I was massaging her feet. I think subconsciously she was preparing to die and to move into a separated space. I remember that very well.

Did you talk to each other about death?

No. Not at all. Two days before she died she called Father and me into the sitting room and said, 'I want a small funeral and I want the slow movement of Mozart's Clarinet Concerto.' That was the only time she ever acknowledged that she was going to die. I think this attitude fitted with her life, she couldn't name her emotional experiences, which brings me back to trying to understand my own depression this year. I was very nurtured as a child but because my parents couldn't name feelings easily, I also grew up in a slight emotional void. Despite the warmth and love, any narrative of negative feelings just didn't exist. Perhaps I have answered that question – when I am with someone who is going through intensely difficult experiences and who is in distress – it is not that I talk about myself but I am sitting there as someone who has some insight. Even though I cannot 'know' anybody else's pain, I can become more myself with someone, more completely and more deeply, when I am sharing in their suffering. That was so special with my mother when she was dying.

Listening to you now it makes me think that psychiatry is going to win out as your specialty over general practice. For one thing you are so interested in narrative and you are also highly attuned to *listening* to the body in pain.

What I want to be able to do with my life is to become more and more adept at being able to imagine other people's realities and engage with the voices that want to communicate with the doctor. It's what you try to do when someone is telling you that they feel ill. Doctors who have suffered themselves are less likely to be arrogant in the face of others' suffering, I hope.

For me it is also critical to be aware of the person who is sitting opposite me. Patterns of breathing – what is their breath doing? What is mine doing? Are we synchronized... what part of the body is the breath coming from...? You said earlier that you were your mother's advocate in her illness and I am wondering whether you were also able to act as a guide in her death?

The day she died she got up in the morning. By then she had a bed in the sitting room as she had been sleeping on the sofa until the district nurse arranged it. She died with a beautiful view of her garden. We put her bed under a photograph of the Himalayas; the setting was perfect. It was a very sunny day at

329

the end of April and I had sent my father out to play golf for respite. She got up for five minutes and then she went back to bed. Our GP came to visit us at lunchtime and talked to both of us, as she was aware that unconscious people still hear. I just lay on the sofa for hours and watched my mother sleeping. Her last words to me were spoken on the previous night when she told me how much I meant to her. She went to sleep and she didn't ever wake up again. My concern had been that my mother would wake up in terrible pain and we wouldn't be able to get any help. Remember, I was not a medic then. I felt very exposed as it was too late to get a Macmillan nurse and I knew that I was alone in the night with my mother slipping away. People often die when their loved ones have left the room. Maybe the dying can't let go easily if their loved ones are sitting beside them as they don't want to cause more pain. It was very important to me that she didn't die alone so my father and I just sat beside her the whole day and evening. I kept telling her to go to sleep and that I would stay by her as I was trying to give her permission to die. In fact the moment before someone dies they often wake up because they have this huge rush of adrenaline, which might even be the origin of the white tunnel experience. The dying will often wake up at the moment before death and open their eyes and my mother did just that. I said, 'It's all okay, you can rest now and sleep.'

I sat with her body for two hours but I didn't want her to go cold in the house – that is my only regret – that I didn't wait until the morning to have her body taken away. I hadn't thought about it much before, but her body was taken away too soon for me. I suspect that the memory of the young man in South Africa, whose dead body was the first I ever witnessed, traumatized me. I visited his body three weeks after he had died and it had changed during the time it took to travel back in the heat to the village where he was to be buried. There was an element of horror for me as I filed past his body with the elders who were all weeping. His face was transformed in death. I wanted to remember my mother warm and alive. In the middle of the night the undertakers came and covered her body with a white sheet. Only then I dissolved. After the body had gone I became fixated on the fact that I hadn't brushed her hair before she left. When I came down the next morning I found her glasses on the table by her bed. Her death was a huge event for me, and now I realize that I hadn't separated from her before she died, although I had been so independent but then I discovered that I hadn't ever emotionally separated from her.

Now, I am beginning to see that the depression I was diagnosed with at the end of May is not only about my grief for Billy, but also about my mother. Five months after she died I forced myself out of bed and went to medical school and became a 'nobody' in an anonymous and hierarchical institution. I gave up my professional status and started from the bottom all over again.

You didn't feel at all special at medical school among all those 'beginners' even when you already had so much life experience to call upon?

No, I wasn't 'special' any more in the way I had been in my other career. That anonymity came as a relief. Yes, I felt special in the way I felt alienated from the others around me but I kept my head below the parapets and just did my work. Then, after the third year of my six-year degree I had Isaac and we had to deal with his illness.

DOCTORS DISSECTED

In some ways I am imagining that it must have enhanced the loss of your mother.

Absolutely. I felt that the melancholy had worsened a year or two after she had died. I don't think many people understand that it can take time for the devastation of loss to set in, and my family also fragmented after her death. I remember getting on a tube after she died and I felt like I was tripping again on acid, my reality was so altered, and yet nobody knew and they were all just getting on with their own lives.

Despite the depression, it seems you were able to cope with medical school.

I could. I functioned as a depressive for several years and the same thing happened this year when, after my nephew Billy died, I was in absolute despair and just wanted to disappear under my duvet and not come out at all except for Isaac and for my brother and sister-in-law.

After my mother died, my next experience of seeing dead bodies was at the medical school a few months later where, as a pre-med, I had to do chemistry and physics. We didn't yet go routinely into the human dissecting rooms. One day we were invited into this room where all the tables were covered in human heads, yes ten disembodied human heads. Different medical schools have different systems and we learnt from dissecting sections rather than working on entire corpses. I walked in and there were ten heads in front of me in this cold and clinical room with its polished shiny surfaces and bright lights. I walked in with a group of 18-year-olds; there had been absolutely no preparation for our brutal introduction to death. I had a visceral reaction, as I was sitting on a high stool, trying to focus, and I remember looking down at the shiny floor and thinking that was a long way down as I became faint and dizzy. Being so recently bereaved I just kept thinking that these decapitated heads were people with histories and families who loved them. Then, we had a lecture from a forensic pathologist, which involved showing us slides of the most awful murder and suicide scenes and dead babies, all of which have become eternally engraved on my mind. A friend at another medical school told me that they did have whole bodies for dissection but they weren't allowed to look at the heads, which had to remain covered throughout the dissections. I find that equally distasteful.

When we were talking last week, you said that for a short while, the depression lifted on the train while you celebrated the universe and life – has that changed this week? You don't strike me as someone who is suffering from a clinical depression as I listen to you so engaged in our dialogue. I feel such a strong life force as you speak to me.

Well, looking after Isaac has been the absolute light of my life. I loved having a tiny baby and being in the moment of this tiny dependent thing but I shall always be bereaved. When Billy died I was with him, with my brother and sister-in-law, and that week – seeing their distress – was the worst trauma that I have ever experienced. Afterwards, I had to take six weeks off work because I couldn't function. When I went back to work, on an adult Cardiology ward I did my best for my patients but I found myself not caring. I just kept thinking, 'They have lived 60, 70 years, they have had a life.'

How could you focus? It feels to me that what you have been through would overthrow anyone. How could you withstand the pain of so much loss and trauma?

I completely crashed, although I put on a face for my child. I've been good at putting a face on but I was filled with self-blame and I started self-medicating with alcohol. There is a history of that in my family and for the first time I had to say to myself, 'This is what depression feels like,' and I have been firefighting it for a long time. Losing Billy was catastrophic and I could no longer live my life in the same way. I wanted to see the GP who knew all about my neonatal experience with Isaac but she wasn't available. I decided then that I had to try medication, as I was too far down not to consider trying it. It was in May, when I was working on the Surgical ward. It was so hard to get up in the morning but once on the ward it was okay and I knew I could lose my own pain when I was needed to look after others' pain. It was the Colorectal ward we have spoken about and that can be intense and medically challenging. There were young women there of my age who had had huge bowel surgery, and women with cervical cancer, which had gone to their bowel. There were stoma bags to manage and very difficult interventions to be made but I did find it rewarding and I was working with the most fantastic registrar. She knew what was going on in my life and in fact she was the only doctor I have ever been able to share anything massive with, my personal doctor friends excluded.

I think that people reading your account might think, 'But how could she not be depressed?' It is not as though it has descended from nowhere but in response to what you have been called upon by 'fate' to live through. Having studied Classics you are probably far more aware than most of the

334

OH! THERE IS SO MUCH I COULD SPEAK ABOUT DEATH

Aristotelian ideas of tragedy whereby the action has to be about something significant enough to make the audience feel pity for the character. Of course pity is not a word with good associations in our modern idiom, but it was used differently then, and it was also required for the audience to fear whether or not the character will be able to survive the blows of his destiny. Recognition also plays a very important part in Greek drama and in your case it has not been so much in recognizing the consequences of hidden actions, as Oedipus has to, but in recognizing your own emotional limitations.

Absolutely, Jane, and there is a sort of paradox here as my therapist has said to me, this depression has come out of my life's circumstances and I have also lost a very complicated pregnancy which we have not had time to talk about. I don't think depression just comes out of the blue, but it comes out of life.

I agree in your context but I also think that one of the most awful depressions to witness is an endogenous depression, which may overtake somebody whose life seems to exist in a harmonious external context and even to be enviable. I know lots of lives that look enviable from the outside but when you burrow beneath the surface it is proved not to be the case. I have also known people for whom one can find no conscious explanation for their depression. I am then left wondering whether they have not been privy to secrets in the family matrix, perhaps a stillborn sibling has preceded their birth, or some trans-generational suffering that has never been verbally disclosed. So yes, I have to agree that there probably is always a reason even if it isn't accessible to conscious thought.

335

On the other hand, I remember the GP saying to me at the end of the consultation, 'How do you want me to categorize this?' Doctors have to categorize every consultation. There is depressive disorder, non-specific mood disorder and many other euphemisms, and I said, 'Oh just put down depression.' I owned and inhabited it that day, which I should have done a long time ago. The other point of the paradox is that if you have these experiences in life they take away your sense of safety. I convinced myself a while ago, for example, that I had ovarian cancer and would be ripped away from Isaac, and so my sense of safety that I have taken for granted since I was a child has been completely destroyed. Now, I see its destruction to be part of the state of growing up and I can observe the world as it really is, full of suffering.

Yes, I have always felt that children who lose a parent prematurely are changed forever and that safety net, which is so important in being able to take life for granted is irreparably torn away. Losing a parent as an adult can be a life-changing experience too, but it does follow the expected trajectory, whereas losing a child is an unspeakable thing.

I think the first 20 years of my life were golden, and then my innocence was shattered when I witnessed the poverty and disease I encountered in the South African townships, but not even that prepared me for the terrors that were waiting for me in my thirties. So, yes, that is why I feel most at ease when I am with people who are enduring catastrophe. I feel that is where I want to be, and although GPs play a crucial role with complex and interesting patients, they also have to deal with a lot of minor illness and I wouldn't be as good at that. Medicine has promised so much to so many people. I don't always see now what medicine offers – apart from crucial progress made in the basics like antibiotics, safe childbirth, safe water and surgery – yes surgeons save lives. If you look at the evidence for chemotherapy, for example, you could argue that it is a bit of a myth. I think there are a lot of doctors who would refuse it, if they had an advanced and complicated cancer. Lance Armstrong was cured of his testicular cancer by chemo but that is exceptional because testicular cancer is very chemo-sensitive, but if you look at the statistics of all survival rates it is really marginal.

I have often thought of chemotherapy being rather like the witch doctor's broth, and a huge experiment on the human animal at best.

Sometimes I feel I am the only one who can see the emperor has got no clothes on. Even with the sophisticated technology and trappings of Intensive Care, beneath the lights and constant measuring, they are often actually only doing basic things, like giving fluids. Medicine needs to come off its pedestal. I don't want to say I have become cynical but I have become 'seeing'. If I think of the most satisfying clinical encounters I have had over the last 15 months, they have been in 'being' with people. Nothing to do with their bodies but just sitting with patients who are in hospital for surgery and finding the time to listen. I have sat on the Oncology ward with my mother, I have been on the trolley myself, and had complex genetic investigations without getting any answers. I have been on that side of the medical fence and understand how vulnerable people are. I can see it in their eyes, but you have to want to look. In the frontline of NHS work, this human vulnerability easily gets lost, but we are always dealing with people and not just their bodies. I feel myself straddling two worlds but, first and foremost, I am an advocate for my patients, which means that I am a challenging Junior Doctor and one who

337

is not afraid of authority and remains unimpressed by medical power. I have been changed forever by the awfulness of seeing a child I loved die suddenly.

16
EACH OF US IS MERELY A SMALL INSTRUMENT

July 2013

I am due to spend the day with Martin; we have not met often over the summer during which time I have been anxious about him. When we last met in late June he did not look at all well. How could the Martin who always arrived in my room like a tornado of energy have changed into a hollow and ill looking man? At that time, although he had lost visible weight and had a constant low fever, his symptoms did not have any name. Now, we have almost reached the end of our book, my writer's block has dissolved and much has happened to both of us, and to our bodies, that we could not have predicted. We must be grateful that what might have become a terminal diagnosis for Martin has, after weeks of investigation and uncertainty, been identified as a chronic and debilitating autoimmune disease, rather than lymphoma, from which Martin is now making a slow and challenging recovery.

I have not been alone in my anxieties as we share several patients in common who – on finding Martin to be on uncertain sick leave from his surgery, with uncontained rumours abounding – arrive in my room teary eyed and anxious on three counts. They are anxious because of Martin's sudden indisposition, a lack of information and more selfishly for this unexpected absence of their trusted and beloved doctor.

DOCTORS DISSECTED

Okay, shall we have just 60 seconds on my illness? Although my medical history looks quite dramatic each one of the previous four events have been something surgical, and even the kidney donation only required five days in hospital, and six weeks off work. They were all a matter of mechanics, of what I call nuts and bolts. Then, this summer getting an illness where I lost weight, had night sweats, overall weakness and to begin with thought I had a 'flu-like virus.

I ignored the symptoms for eight or nine weeks, although I was losing weight and having night sweats. Then, I took my own bloods and they were all normal, which reassured me for a bit. But I couldn't escape the fact that I was getting worse, especially with atypical exhaustion and so I reluctantly went to see a consultant physician who specializes in difficult diagnoses, the 'physicians' physician', Dr Paul Glynne at University College Hospital. Very unusually, Cosmo was so worried that he insisted on coming with me. Paul Glynne took 17 tubes of blood – normally taking even four or five is quite a lot and he did a CT scan of my chest and abdomen, which was normal. He diagnosed a postviral syndrome. Six or seven weeks later, by now we are in July, I had lost several more kilos in weight and had to return to Dr Glynne. He said, 'You don't lose this kind of weight with postviral syndromes and you must now have a PET scan, a colonoscopy, an endoscopy and we need to take more bloods.' The bloods were all normal but the PET scan showed a multiplicity of PET avid lymph nodes throughout my chest, and we then needed a biopsy, so Paul referred me to a chest physician who did a bronchoscopy.

That is a horrid procedure isn't it?

Not nice. He went through the wall of the bronchus into the mediastinum and got a biopsy of my lymph nodes. It wasn't too bad, you remember shady bits of it, but it wasn't really an ordeal. Then there was the uncomfortable wait for the diagnosis of sarcoidosis.* For the first time in my life I had an illness, which could have a difficult outcome, or it might grind on interminably.

At one stage there was a fear that it was lymphoma wasn't there?

When you have got all those nodes it is either sarcoidosis, lymphoma, TB, or a chronic lymphatic leukaemia. A lot of suspense was riding for me on the horse of that biopsy. There was the additional irony that I have got a fabulous Critical Illness insurance policy so if it had have been a lymphoma, which in many presentations can be curable, I would have been ill but fabulously rich! However, it was sarcoidosis, and probably it is the best of the options, because most people have recovered in two years. Now, I am taking 30mgs of prednisolone a day, and tomorrow it will be reduced to 20mgs for the next four weeks, and then another PET scan.

Is that a high dosage?

Yes, the usual dose is between 5–7mgs a day. Of course, there are lots of side effects; it is a bit like taking an amphetamine, it is speedy stuff. Very quickly, within a week, I was feeling much better, and walking better, because the problem is the fatigue

---

* Sarcoidosis is a chronic multisystem disorder which defies full understanding: there are symptoms of fatigue, malaise, anorexia, weight loss and some respiratory symptoms. Exaggerated T helper CD4 lymphocyte responses are involved with the possibility that there is a cellular immune response damaging the body tissues of the patient, leading to disease in joints, lung, heart, eyes and liver with a widespread but variable degree of involvement in different individuals.

and the weakness, which had cut me back to 200 yards. I knew I had to stop work when I couldn't any more manage the stairs to my office and I would have to sit down and recover before calling up a patient, which was only a week before last. Anyway, I am hoping to go back to work part-time on the 7 October but I will decide nearer the time. I am doing an ethics course at Imperial College at the end of September, so that will be a litmus test. Today, I walked here from Baker Street, which was probably five hundred yards, without any difficulty.

As ever, you are very good at providing a medical history but one that is unaccompanied by your feelings. Do you contemplate on how seriously ill you are?

I have. I was also very low in spirit because – first of all – I felt that people, that my colleagues, thought I was putting it on a bit; they clearly don't know me. And, also, people thought I had depression. Postviral syndrome would also be a terrible diagnosis to have, rather like IBS. Imagine me getting myalgic encephalopathy, when it has been such a puzzle to me as a doctor to understand the mechanics of that diagnosis throughout my career. Sarcoidosis mimics the symptoms of postviral diseases but it is a scientific diagnosis. I have often thought my patients had depression rather than a truly immunological condition, which is still the focus of an academic and medical battleground. Even Simon Wessely, the Professor of Psychiatry, who has focused his career on postviral illness, has abandoned his research into postviral syndromes because he has been made the victim of a brigade of people – rather like the hunt saboteurs – who hate anyone who talks about it being partially, or fully, a psychological illness. He is the expert that has promoted a return to graded physical exercise and Cognitive Behavioural Therapy as a treatment plan, which immediately suggests to most people that postviral is of a dreaded psychiatric origin.

In your case you went to the physicians' physician, Dr Glynne, or sarcoidosis might not have been diagnosed.

Yes. And that is what worries me, the number of people out there who don't have the privilege of access to all of those invasive and very expensive investigations, which were completed in my case in three weeks. Whereas, if you live in Clitheroe or Penzance, you are likely to be put on antidepressants. There will be hundreds of people in that situation and now, with hindsight, that has become very upsetting to me.

Presumably, most of them will get better in two years, but by then many of them will also have lost their jobs, or their relationships and their lives will fall apart. Even now I reckon I am not out of the woods yet because it has been a very stormy and difficult time, and yet I have had a diagnosis, which may not have happened if I lived anywhere other than London.

Earlier in our meetings you said that you want to live to be 99 and that your worst fear is getting Alzheimer's, like your father, except that you have religiously observed a healthy lifestyle. When you got ill…

I thought how you never know what is waiting for you around the next corner and you have got to live absolutely for 'now!' because for the first time in my life, even today, I'm thinking, 'Oh God! I have got a diagnosis, I have an illness, I now have a chronic label.' I have got to get over it and I probably will, but it is a sobering thought. I have realized that, although I am

343

thin and wiry and eat the right things, I am as vulnerable as the next person and I might be struck down and not, after all, live to be 92. As I have said elsewhere my greatest fear is to get a dementing illness, particularly as my memory is hopeless, but now my mortality has been heightened. In the last six months I have thought a lot about my patients who have died; particularly when I drive past their houses or come across conditions, which provoke transient thoughts about the conditions that they have died from. In fact, most of them have not died from cancer. I have been thinking a lot about death. As you grow older as a GP, your cohort of patients grows older with you and you are then seeing people who have grown up with you over the last 25 years and are now entering the end-of-life category.

When you think about your mortality, what do you feel?

I feel contented; although if I found that I had something lethal I would be disappointed that I had been swindled out of certain things that are still on my shopping list to do. I have still got ambitions, I would like to finish this book, they are quite mundane but there are things I want to read and to travel more, not to exotic destinations, but in the UK. I am off to the Isle of Lewis this weekend and I want to learn about navigation and to learn to sail and cope with my boat without an instructor. To be brave at sea, go through the Caledonian Canal, and on to France. As you know I have brought a boat, quite a big boat, along with Rachel and I want to become a master of the sea.

As you will know better than me when illness takes hold of the body all the libido or energy, I don't of course just mean sexual, is drawn back into the self. As a doctor, or rather the

kind of doctor you are, who is so immediately available, still so passionate to respond, even when you are tired, I am trying to imagine what it might have felt like when illness rendered you incapable. I know you are too sensible to think of yourself as indispensable, but when forces greater than oneself overtake there can also be a loss of status and a sense of infantilization.

Yes, it truncated everything. I felt that I was not so much losing my touch medically but I had to cut down on everything I did. I knew that the penalty for not doing that could be serious; not bothering as much, which can lead to mistakes. It didn't last long, but for the two months when I did not have a diagnosis I couldn't work out how to stop. There was no reason to stop working except that I didn't feel well, but that was just too vague. I am always carrying a great vapour of unresolved problems and an overweight in-tray. Even now, as I sit here, one of my colleagues, a senior Consultant Neurologist, needs his 360-degree appraisal doing, and it cannot be delayed any longer. I am supposed to sort out all the forms and fill in the endless boxes. I will get around to it in a day or two but that does not fit well with someone who likes to be meticulous, to be up-to-date, to be reliable and always to be the guy to ask. Yes, I have had to abandon all that and it feels strange and unsatisfactory and, even with my PA, I couldn't manage. Every day Elaine, my PA for the last 25 years, would say, 'How are you?' And I would reply, 'Not very well.' We didn't know what to do about it.

Yes, I know because when I saw you, you would have a clammy forehead and you looked green, which even now is only being controlled by the prednisolone and which brings me to another observation. Doctors seem very poor at acknowledging illness in each other. It is as though they are dealing with it so much

that, when it is sitting in front of them, they turn a blind and dangerous, even a mocking and unkind, eye to each other. They can be very unkind.

I think it is both true and odd, and one explanation is that we all tend to run into our office and get on with the day's work. We don't have a forum, not even a water cooler we can gather around, in our practice, and so it is possible for things to go unnoticed…

Sorry, that is a bit of a feeble excuse when just one sight of you has been enough to send a shiver down my spine.

Well, it is a bit of an excuse. Another component is that there is a tacit agreement that doctors do not get ill. We are doctors and not patients and so we are on the other side of the Berlin Wall. We carry on, that is what we do. We do not get illnesses, but perhaps people were just nervous about approaching me.

And is that how you would behave?

I would like to think now I wouldn't, that I have learnt something from this experience, but I think I might have done so before. I have sometimes been very careless about things that my colleagues have shared with me. I think, looking back, that I may have been harsh and thoughtless, and when colleagues have said, 'It's fine,' even though I could see it was far from fine, I didn't do anything about it.

When we last met before the diagnosis was made, you were in such a state that your professional reappraisal wasn't going to

go through and now I am wondering if what then seemed to me to be irrational anxiety about a forgone conclusion was exacerbated by the way you were still undiagnosed and without a label, but feeling anxious about yourself and your health? It seemed so strange that you had such a dip in confidence when you also had recently been made one of the few GPs in private general practice to become a Fellow of the Royal College of GPs?

That is true, but those persecutory forms had to be in by 1 June. I was already late and had already been fined £500 for being late. The problem was that a bureaucratic demand was being made for so much material, as there are 16 or 18 paragraphs of what I consider to be irrelevant data to be filled in. For example, one of the paragraphs is 'Probity'.

Sorry, what does probity mean?

That you are ethical in a financial sense, that you do not do anything nefarious like getting commissions for ordering imaging scans, or favour certain medications because of financial remuneration. There are other things that you have got to present, like letters of criticism or complaint. You have got to declare if there have been any complaints at all and give your analysis of each of them, however petty and time wasting they are. You have got to present and list each of the postgraduate activities that you have undertaken but, even more than that, you have got to show how these postgraduate activities have affected your current practice. Your appraiser then looks at all your documentation. You have an annual appraisal, which can last for three hours with your appraisal officer. When five years' worth of appraisals are collated, the officer then instructs the General Medical Council as to whether you are fit to be re-licensed, or not, for another five years. I am going to be re-licensed in December but my appraisal officer had got on to me and told me that I had not uploaded enough documentation. The reasons I hadn't were multifold: I was kicking out about uploading on to the computer because it is very time-heavy and every document has to be scanned and then uploaded and I didn't understand the system. Every time I tried, the password had changed, and there are several different passwords for different components of the system. Meantime, I am trying to deal with my patients, their emails, and management issues, my colleagues, and not feeling well, feeling nauseous. And, finally I find myself going to the loo to throw up between patients. Meantime, I am trying to upload all the data, which was just the last straw on the camel's back, and then I receive a warning that I have not done enough. I forced myself to rally and spent several half days at it. I uploaded so much stuff – I wanted to swamp them – and put everything in that I had written, including the *Daily Mail* articles, so it was three or four thousand hours of work and research in a year. I thought, 'That will show them.' The appraiser was very impressed with me and now I have another five more years' license but you still have to do the annual appraisal or to be struck off. It is a complete shift in thinking which has come in on the back of the Harold Shipman scandal. Everyone agrees he would have passed with flying colours; he was marvellous academically and everyone also thought he was a terrifically attentive doctor.

I thought you sounded in a panic at that time…

No, not panic, but I was angry at having this foisted upon me at this late stage in my career. I think it is fine when it is introduced to someone like Cosmo while he is moving up the ranks because he is familiar with it, because he and his friends already have a system that whenever they do anything at all, they immediately upload it on to the Internet in readiness. They live their whole lives filling in their files. It is a bit like always trying to please 'sir', but I am not wired like that. Cosmo says, 'Dad, every time I read an article in the BMJ, I enter it into my file automatically.' I am not wired to running my life or professional development like that. Cosmo was trained throughout university to tick every box as he went along but we were not. We were trained, 'To see one, do one, teach one.'

Talking to Cosmo last week, I said, 'How are you finding doing Anaesthetics at West Middlesex Hospital?' He told me that he had had to go to a cardiac arrest in a small child on his first day and he had never done a paediatric one before and that fazed him. Whereas, when he was at Charing Cross in the Intensive Therapy Unit, he was learning how to put in a long line [a thin catheter inserted into an artery] using an ultra- sound scanner to position it in the right place. Before he had completed that course, been examined in it and ticked the box, he was still allowed to put a long line in any other way. Now that he has successfully learnt the technique, he is not allowed to do it in any other way. The technique has become that orchestrated, yes that regulated, which worries me.

Are there other ways to put a line in?

Yes, yes the way we used to do it: tip them upside down, look for a vein and shove it in and if that doesn't work you try the other side. That is how you develop a range of clinical skills. It is like learning to make a soufflé. Imagine, only learning to make a soufflé in one way and then once you have been examined in it and the recipe box is ticked, you are never allowed to explore another recipe.

DOCTORS DISSECTED

That takes us back to the beginning of the book when Dr Holden describes being outside of the BMA when the explosion occurred and his broadcast about how today's doctors have become too specialized in their trainings.

Today's headlines in the *Daily Mail* are that only five consultant A&E doctors are actually inside of hospitals during the night across the nation. Yes, they may be on call at home but they are not there on the hospital site and that is not the same thing at all. We need to have really experienced people on Casualty, doctors who have seen it all and not newly qualified doctors.

You mentioned that when you last talked to Cosmo he appealed to you to see the many improvements in the NHS as well as the disappointments.

Yes, and I can see the good side too. What I am irritated about is how they have hijacked the word 'reflective'. Everything now is about 'reflective practice' and the people who have designed the appraisal have got the wrong word. It should not be about 'reflective practice' but about 'meta-cognition', when you think internally about certain things and you learn and profit from your process. 'Reflective' is a more lightweight word and it annoys me that it crops up on every page of the appraisal. I feel people who are not adept at what a doctor's postgraduate professional development should be have put the whole appraisal process together. What frustrates me is that every time I see a patient – and I probably do 50 interactions a day, from prescribing eye drops for someone with an allergy to dealing with somebody who has crushing central chest pain – all the time, I am thinking, 'Are these the right eye drops? What will they cost him? Are they the best ones for allergy? Is it an allergy?' All the time you are

EACH OF US IS MERELY A SMALL INSTRUMENT

reflecting on what you do and to be asked to substantiate on what you do makes me think that the person asking the questions does not understand my daily tasks. I am not interested in playing the game academically or politically.

The Royal College of General Practitioners was only founded in 1952, whereas Henry VIII founded my main college, the Royal College of Physicians. You at least have a sense of history there and the greatest doctors that have ever practised have all had Membership. In Henry's reign health care was in a mess, well there was not any health care; there were people shoving herbs and there were alchemists and quacks. It was all very confused and the Age of Enlightenment had not arrived. Henry had a fantastic administration, which had the sense to try and impose some order on the medical profession as documented in a painting by Holbein, which we could go and see. The men in the painting are all named and we know what they did. It is called Holbein's Cartoon, and it is displayed at the Royal College of Surgeons. As I was saying the physicians ground physic, in other words, herbs, thought to be curative, and today at the College of Physicians there is a beautiful herb garden that is worth a visit and they also had links ultimately with the Chelsea Physic Garden. Their duty was to try and stamp out quackery but most of it was quackery, because science as we know it now did not exist and the microscope had not been invented. There was a growing sense that the profession of physicians was evolving from apprenticeship and with less status were the barber surgeons. It was only much later that the universities got involved in training doctors on the back of the royal colleges, which were offering qualifications until the twentieth century. Then the universities started to appoint qualifications and the royal colleges became relegated to postgraduate institutions.

In the middle of the 20th century, around the time of the Second World War, physicians wore two hats and functioned

351

both inside of hospitals and outside in the community. It was only after the war that family doctors, or GPs, were now only in the community and the doctors who worked in the hospitals – who were physicians and not surgeons – began to specialize and to become Cardiologists or Chest Physicians, or whatever. By 1952 we had the formation of the Royal College of GPs, and Family Medicine became the icon of the NHS. In other countries, people did not have family doctors, as it was a concept that was created by the NHS. Prior to war, family doctors would have their panel and people paid four and sixpence a year to be under the care of a particular doctor.

Some of those pre-war GPs became very famous. There was a man called Will Pickles who practised from a bungalow at Aysgarth in the Yorkshire Dales, which I have been to see. Pickles, for example, documented, which is now known to the world, the incubation periods for measles, infectious hepatitis and mumps. He put all those things on the map without using a laboratory but only by using coloured drawing pins to make graphs. He knew through hearsay who had met whom at each country fair and how so and so got that illness from somebody else. Today, there is an annual Will Pickles Memorial Lecture, which I like to go to. I've made a pilgrimage to his house because, all over the world, everybody knows what he accomplished without any laboratory tests.

Despite your frustrations with the ways NHS medicine is evolving is there anything that you envy about Cosmo's skills and training?

Well, now he is doing very high technical things. I would love to have all those skills, because I am a craft sort of person who loves using their hands and you lose all those skills. Secondly, with modern techniques and training and so on there are so many opportunities to do sophisticated medical things. I also miss the camaraderie and bantering of other skilled people such as Caroline was talking about: the uniqueness of being in Theatre as part of a team. And you know how much I deeply resent my paperwork. I think Cosmo has had a better academic training than I had because it has been more formal; I envy him that. I look back and justify myself by reminding myself how often my consultant colleagues will ring me for advice. I told you about my eye consultation last Friday when the consultant hijacked my consultation for himself.

Was going to the eye doctor another anxiety about this illness and your fear of declining vision?

Yes, I thought the steroids were giving me a cataract. I waited for four weeks to see the consultant privately because he was so heavily booked. I landed up in front of the great man and I told him about my sarcoidosis and how I was worried about my eyesight and he said, 'No, no, just a moment. I have got a very swollen lip,' pointing just under his nose at the philtrum. 'It has swollen up overnight and I'm really worried about what it might be, what do you think it is?' I had a look and said, 'What have you been up to, have you been working in the garden at dusk, or anything?' He told me that he had washed his car last night and I said, 'I think it is an insect bite,' which it was. I told him to get on to the pharmacy and take 10mgs of prednisolone right away. Fortunately, my own anxieties about my eyes were ill-founded and they are fine.

Oh, I haven't spoken about becoming a grandfather to Cosmo's daughter. At the naming of Thea, I was very moved when Cosmo gave a little speech; he got so tearful that he had to stop and I think the reason was how his grandfather was missing. It was very interesting because Cosmo never reveals any emotions, as you know, but he couldn't go on speaking and Cecilie had to step in.

You don't think there was a different reason, because he has told me that he never thinks about his grandfather, so I have a different take on it. Perhaps his tears were for you, and seeing you standing there not with your usual buoyancy but fragile.

He did also say he wanted to preface the day by remembering people who couldn't be there.

Yes, but I really don't think that would make Cosmo well up with tears.

Well, maybe he is worried that there is another grandfather who is going to pop off. It is true my father was no better a grandfather than he was a father, as he never communicated with anyone. Cosmo has also been concerned about Ben. Shall I tell you what has happened about Ben's kidney?

Do you mean after Cosmo's wedding when he had to come back to London and go straight on to dialysis?

Yes. His kidney function started to dramatically decline and as his creatinine level markers shot up to five or six hundred – normal would be 120 – he had to go urgently on to dialysis.

EACH OF US IS MERELY A SMALL INSTRUMENT

I think that is what Cosmo dreads – seeing his own creatinine levels going off the page.

It was assumed the Luder-Sheldon kidney gene that he had inherited from Glynis was responsible and that it was just odd that it had suddenly declined, or maybe it was because he was also diabetic. No more thought was given to why it should have happened and he was prepared for a transplantation from Nico his boyfriend. It all took place at the Hammersmith Hospital where the operation was performed by the surgeon Nadey Hakim, who is the wizard transplanter. He also did Glynis's second transplant when he discovered what had happened to the failed first kidney that I donated. They were monitoring Ben post operatively when the new kidney that Nico had given him suddenly started going off the page too, which it should not have done because he was on nice antirejection stuff. It wasn't due to rejection going on as they took biopsies to prove that. Then, they worked out that the kidney had FCGS, which is a form of glomerulonephritis.

I know about nephritis but what is the glomerulus bit about?

Well, glomeruli are the functional units of the kidney. Your kidney is rather like a blackberry, or raspberry and all the little blobs that compose the berry are the little glomeruli and each glomerulus is a little micro-filter that is filtering your blood and creating urine and all the pipes join up. Your kidney is a cluster of all the thousands of glomeruli. Glomerulonephritis happens when they all get inflamed for some reason. It turns out that Ben had another disease that had buggered up his original kidneys and was totally different from his mother's genetic condition, and totally separate from diabetes, but possibly autoimmune, and that disease had now also destroyed Nico's transplanted kidney. The consultants have said that they are going to transplant him again from a corpse and give him a new pancreas as well, to get rid of the diabetes. This time they are going to give him the monoclonal antibody that stops the nephritis before they transplant. They had to go to America to find out how to proceed.

How old is Ben?

1976 he was born, and so he is 37.

Is he up and about?

Oh yes, he is at work. He is incredibly plucky but he is on the edge – just on the cusp of having to go back on to dialysis – which he doesn't want to do but once you start vomiting there is no choice.

He is going to get a new pancreas and kidney, in three months?

Well, the waiting list is four months but anyone needing a double transplant is given priority. Apparently, it is a pretty big operation and the immune-postoperative suppressive dangers are even greater but as ever Ben is putting his best foot forward and jolly glad it is going to happen. I have had a letter at the *Daily Mail* from a woman whose daughter has had it done and she is cured and thrilled. The poignant thing about it is that someone walking about out there has got to die first. They are out there today, at work.

The donor has got to be both young and healthy?

EACH OF US IS MERELY A SMALL INSTRUMENT

Yes, like one of the scaffolders outside of your window falling off the roof, or whatever. Did you hear in the news this week that a woman from, was it Lancaster or York, had had a transplant from a five-week-old baby? The baby died of heart disease and they used his micro kidneys to transplant into a woman.

They grow?

Yes, they grow, apparently they grow to about two-thirds of the size to what they would have reached and the parents gave their permission. It is an interesting new development, and it brings me back to the more optimistic future for Cosmo's baby, Thea, as to whether or not she has got the disease, and when we are going to make the intervention to find out. Cosmo leaves it obscure, as to when he was diagnosed, in his interview, but actually we found out when Glynis was in hospital after she had my kidney in 1992, when he was eight. I thought Cosmo shouldn't know before he had reached the age of reason, which is seven.

Baby Thea…then there is a horrible question as to whether she is carrying the gene? Oh dear!

It is an autosomal dominant gene and so she has got a 50-percent chance. Autosomal means it is not on a sex chromosome but it is on one of your other chromosomes, so men or women can pass it on. Dominant means that half your chromosomes have it and half your sperms have it, which brings the chance up to 50 per cent. Cosmo had a 50-per-cent chance of not getting it but he got it. So that is how it is. There is a thing in genetics called penetrance, which means that you may hold the gene but you may not express it, it is random.

DOCTORS DISSECTED

I don't think it has struck anybody else, and certainly not Cosmo, that I went off creating other children and endlessly trying to justify it to myself because there would then be a bank of kidneys. I don't have any shame about it. All my children, including the two whom I am sadly not in contact with, are fabulous and successful and have been well looked after. I have had several fantastic relationships. It matters to me a lot that I didn't see my marriage through to the end; I wish that had been possible. I would like to have been successful there. I didn't just wander off having other children but the need for kidneys did make it feel better. I am jolly pleased that Cosmo has his options but it means there needs to be more children for Thea. Then again stem cell research may soon provide another solution.

I wonder if knowing all the science is any consolation...do you think that Cosmo, who is already such an academic highflying specialist at 29, is in a very different place to where you were at a similar age?

He certainly has not got the anatomy that we had, or the experiences of dissection. I can sit here and recite to you all about the tiniest duct that comes from your parotid gland, which is positioned along the inside of your cheek, and ends with a little pore in the middle of your cheek that you can feel with your tongue, which is called Stensen's duct. Cosmo might not be able to name it, nor would he think the effort was worthwhile because he would just say, 'If I want to know every duct in the body then I can look them up on the Internet. There is no necessity for me to learn them.' We had all that anatomical and physiological knowledge inside of our heads. Now that Cosmo is studying Anaesthetics, he has become very good at physiology in preparing for the examination. He knows all about pharmacology, and the molecules and the motor end plate, and all of that. When I did my exams for Membership to the Royal College of Physicians, you still had to take it to such a high level in all aspects of physical medicine, so somebody like me has a much broader knowledge base. I could stand up and lecture – even just after qualifying – on impetigo or fulminating pre-eclampsia, but I am a shotgun and Cosmo is a rifle. I learnt and can still recite to you the anatomy of any part of the body, because that is what I had to learn and what I wanted to learn.

What Latin incantation would you like to end our conversation with? I find listening to you is like listening to mysterious poetry.

Scaphoid, lunate, triquetrum, trapezium, trapezoid, capitate, and hamate… Oh, they do not learn all that now, not unless you want to become a wrist surgeon. Today, our young doctors can upload from the Internet anything they want.

Oh! We are, with the random choice of the wrist, back to the beginning of our story and your first viva voce of the forearm and the hand.

17
COSMO BECOMES
A FATHER
(DECEMBER 2013)

Tell me what are the big happenings in your life since we last met, just after you got married in March 2011?

I'm still living in the same place, and obviously, Thea's birth.

No, not obviously Cosmo, as last time we talked you told me that you couldn't imagine how you would be able to fit a baby into your lives. It didn't then seem at all high on your agenda.

The thought that I afterwards shared with Cecilie was that there is never a good time. I read an interesting article the other day about a group of men in their forties who have never married and were now reporting that they wished they had had children. The premise of the article was that they had all waited too long to sort out their careers at the expense of the other things in life. We also thought that there would never be an ideal time, and we would never have enough money to make it easy. It was more me who thought it was a good idea, I always wanted to have children at some point. I couldn't see any reason to leave it any longer because what was going to change?

COSMO BECOMES A FATHER (DECEMBER 2013)

You could only have been 29 when Thea was born and so, all things change all the time.

I also thought Cecilie is older than me and nobody knows how long it is going to take us to get pregnant and I knew she was a bit more hesitant about having children. I also had exams to fit in. We planned that I could do the first part of my Anaesthetic exams – the written part – and then the baby would be born after that. I was still working after Thea was born. I was in a full-time job where I was working very long shifts but at least that meant I could have whole days off in lieu of the shifts.

What's a long day?

A long day is 13 hours. In August, when Thea was two months old, I had another important exam to prepare for, which I took at the beginning of December 2012. The second half of Cecilie's maternity leave has been quite busy with me both working and preparing for another exam and now she's just gone back to work. For the time being different members of the family have been covering for us, and Thea's started with her childminder this week.

How have you felt about becoming a father?

I've quite enjoyed it. I think it's fun and Thea is a very good baby so we are lucky.

Are you opinionated on the subject of child rearing?

I am normally quite opinionated about everything but I seem to be relaxed about Thea. Generally, if she is warm and dry and fed she's fine. I am quite happy to leave her on the sofa, or the bench without surrounding her with pillows the whole time.

On the bench?

Yeah, as long as she is angled correctly so she cannot roll off. Yes, I think I'm quite relaxed and she went to Ikea on her fourth day of life and we travel on the tube with her everywhere.

Do you feel you've been changed at all by becoming a father?

[LONG PAUSE] No, I don't think so; the only words that are coming to me are that I find it fun. Yes, fun is a good word to describe it, but that parenthood is also relentless. The word relentless is neither a good thing nor a bad thing, but it emphasizes that it is continuous. We do often stand there just looking at her. She is very sweet, even hilarious; we also think she's a bit weird, a little oddball. It's fun the way she's always pulling her socks off.

You haven't I imagine had much contact with babies before?

No, so maybe that explains it but I do also think she is a bit weird and quite strange as well. I sometimes feel that she's teasing me but I like to play with her. I don't know how becoming a father has changed me. Is that something people say?

COSMO BECOMES A FATHER (DECEMBER 2013)

Yes, some think the world has changed and other don't. It's a matter of personality type and how much competitive attention the man still needs.

I am trying to work out how much I have changed and how much I am the same but forced to behave differently. I think we still manage to do our own things and I still do my extra bits of teaching and my ambulance work but I gave up doing the lifeboat thing. There is just not enough time, and I do lots of events' medicine and sometimes I earn extra money, but often not.

I am a little confused as to where you now are on your career path and your dad is not great at explaining it to me.

No, he doesn't quite get it, the way it works and for some reason all the colleges are different. For example, the Royal College of Physicians has an exam to become a Medical Registrar, which I now would be if I were training to be a physician. In fact, I wouldn't have any more exams, I would just aim to become a consultant after some more experience and when a vacancy occurred. As an anaesthetist I have two sets of exams: one set to become an Anaesthetic Registrar and another set at the end of the training to exit with the potential for consultant status, which is called the FRCA.

Is Emergency Medicine, which you are also studying in parallel, different again? In fact, hard to believe, but I think you have worked for two unconnected sets of professional exams…

Emergency Medicine requires you to take exams to become a Member of the College of Emergency Medicine and then to sit a later exit exam, which gives you Fellowship to the college and the right to work at consultant level. I have now passed the Membership to Emergency Medicine and Part One of my Fellowship to the Royal College of Anaesthetists as well.

Since becoming a father last June you have now accomplished two major sets of postgraduate exams?

Yes, I've done two big sets of exams, which I was preparing for before Thea's birth and since the ending of 2012. I had to do a huge amount of work for the Anaesthetics examination, where you have to know a huge amount of detail, whereas the Emergency Medicine exam is more clinical and I winged it just a little bit. I crammed in the Emergency exams before Thea was born. I have only just heard this week that I've passed the ones in Anaesthetics and that I can become a registrar. But, then you already know that I am in a rush.

You don't appear to be stressed but I must remind myself how good you are good at concealing your feelings.

It has been a lot of work and it all takes careful planning to fit in going to full-time work, revising, as well as looking after Thea. I am terrible at revising in the evening but that's the only chance I have and Cecilie has had to pick up the slack for the last three months. Obviously, I wanted to pass these exams the first time.

But you know better than me that most people don't.

No, they don't, but I knew that I had to, because I knew Thea was going to be born.

COSMO BECOMES A FATHER (DECEMBER 2013)

I know you are modest but did you pass them well?

Yes, I did.

I know how particular the marking is because one of my clients was doing the equivalent in Oncology and after he retook for the second time, when he had only failed by just one mark, he was told by the university that he wasn't eligible to retake again, but then he appealed. Eventually, after providing medical certificates, he was given dispensation to re-sit, but the stress was horrifying for him to live with. Dare I ask how you passed?

Well, I have sat so many different exams. For example there is the practical one where you go down to the college and sit down at a desk and on the other side are two experienced anaesthetists who question you on anything from the curriculum. They could say, 'Tell me how you anaesthetize a child with Down's syndrome?' or 'You are in A&E and somebody comes in who has been shot – what do you do?' Or, they could say, 'How does an ultrasound machine work?' Or, 'Tell us about the metabolism of morphine.' On that exam I was close to full marks but something that I never learnt threw me. It was my own stupid fault, but I don't know very much about antifungal medicines and I never revised them.

Excuse me, but what is the relevance of antifungal medicine?

I should have known because we cover Intensive Care where people can have severe fungal infections but the reality is that we rarely decide which antifungals to use as it is a specialist microbiology decision. It was the only area I decided not to invest time in, avoiding learning all about the structure of funguses, which are rare. I knew all about bacteria and viruses and how to identify them and which of a thousand different drugs to use but anyway…I was sitting there and they just looked at me and said, 'Tell us about antifungals.' I thought it was a joke, I was hoping it was a joke and I looked at them and said, 'You don't mean antibiotics?' They were surprised as well because everything else they asked me I knew the answer to. I could have done very well.

Come on Cosmo, you did do very well…

Well, I got 45/48.

That is still Distinction isn't it?

Yes, but I've learnt my lesson now. It was my own fault.

And with the Emergency Medicine, how were those exams?

Oh, they were 10 times easier. A lot easier, but they are good exams because if you are any good at Emergency Medicine you are bound to pass the exam, whereas in Anaesthetics, you are supposed to know a huge amount of detail.

There isn't a formal requirement to combine Anaesthetics with Emergency Medicine is there, but if I remember you have your own career agenda, or ambitions.

No. Interestingly, you cannot combine the two professionally: you can do Emergency Medicine and Intensive Care, or you can do Anaesthetics with Intensive Care but you can't do Emergency Medicine with Anaesthetics as a career. As you know, my ambitions are to work with the helicopter emergency services (HEMS) who, unlike in A&E, where you see everything, see only the acute critical care. The fact is that a large part of Emergency Medicine has, with the demise of GPs working out-of-hours, become out-of-hours general practice. I'm not very interested in that. I am interested in anaesthetics, resuscitation, and critical care.

When we last met you still hadn't yet done any anaesthetic procedures unsupported.

No. Now it's more common for me to begin the procedure on my own and then for someone to turn up to join me, but I have done about 15 routine anaesthetics entirely unsupported, and have given over 500 in total, which have all been at the West Middlesex Hospital. At the moment I am trying to develop my paediatric anaesthesia skills, which I find I am becoming more and more interested in.

What is it like having the responsibility to put somebody's child to sleep and then to wake them up?

It's, hmm, I don't know. I wonder if I might specialize in Paediatrics, I sort of enjoy it. Waking up is often more critical and dangerous than the induction of anaesthesia. Children can be quite agitated when they wake up and sometimes you have to hold them so they don't jump off the trolley and hurt themselves. Yes, they are also quite funny and very, very sweet.

DOCTORS DISSECTED

Oh, I am so pleased to hear you don't adopt the same rather cavalier attitude as with Thea on the bench! But what is there to enjoy?

Well, it is definitely a little bit stressful, mostly because you have to hold so many different things in your mind, but it is wonderful to be able to reassure a little child. If I have children on my list, I will go and see the child early because we don't want them hanging around and getting more stressed and scared waiting for their surgery. You have to read their notes and then you have to talk to the parents on a kind of grown-up and give-them-confidence level, while at the same time you have to talk to and play with a little child. It is difficult because they might only be three-years-old and you want to play with them to earn their trust quickly, but at the same time you need to get the past medical history from the parents, who will be even more anxious. There is a lot of information to be gathered and shared. You need to liaise with the nursing staff who may be brilliant, or maybe less able to help. It is difficult but it is also satisfying, and it is quite nice because I like kids and I enjoy the play and the challenge of distracting them.

Although you said earlier that things don't change I see this as a big change in you Cosmo, your growing interest in children, and your wish to try and put them at their ease in very distressing circumstances.

Yes, it is all quite new to me and I find I am enjoying it very much.

Do you ever think about Thea when you are preparing a child?

COSMO BECOMES A FATHER (DECEMBER 2013)

Well, it is interesting as I have had two big paediatric emergencies that I have dealt with since Thea's birth. We got called down to see a baby that was unwell in the Emergency Department. She was a five-month-old girl who was exactly the same age as Thea, even the same weight, who had meningitis. She was very unwell and we had to put lines in and put her to sleep on a ventilator so that she could be transferred to a hospital with Paediatric Intensive Care, which was both disturbing and interesting. She was the youngest child I had ever anaesthetized, as in my routine elective work we don't do anything under one year. Later on we were relieved to hear that she had recovered.

You say that you are chilled and not anxious generally with Thea but does an incident like that affect you personally and leave you with anxiety?

I don't know what you mean by anxiety because I can't do anything about it if Thea were to become seriously ill, but I would be very anxious if she did. I am probably less anxious as a father because although I am relatively inexperienced I do know more than a layperson. I know when a baby is properly unwell – not nearly as much as my dad knows because he's had a lifetime of seeing babies both when they are unwell and well – but I am starting to recognize when a baby is unwell. Thea, touch wood, hasn't been unwell and I have only taken her temperature twice, but mainly because Cecilie wanted me to. I am not a worried father. That's not to say that I wouldn't be scared if Thea had to have an anaesthetic.

Gwen, whom I interviewed earlier said it spooked her when the anaesthetist asked her if she wanted to give her little son a 'final kiss' before he went 'under'.

369

I have thought about that because some anaesthetists do say that when putting children to sleep and I've wondered for that very reason, but you can interpret anything in almost any way.

Is it more stressful anaesthetising children than adults?

You of course have to keep them safe and it is a little bit stressful because things can go wrong very quickly. Yes, the whole thing is more stressful because it is newer to me but I don't have to do it on my own yet. Anaesthetizing a child on my own would be very stressful but, like anything, experience makes it less so.

Have you developed your own style yet?

I think so, a little bit; I am starting to even with the kids. All anaesthetists work alongside an operating-department practitioner and often I've had the same one working with me who is very experienced and has seen a great deal in her time assisting in Theatre. I ask for her opinion as I think it is always useful. She said the other day, 'That's what Cosmo likes,' and we had a conversation about how I've developed my own style in a small way. The way I distract the children, the order I do things. Yes, you experiment with what seems to work. You put that instrument out of sight, and you are still showing them the storybook as you administer the dose, or I might put the blanket on in a certain way to be sure they are warm. I am learning all the time those little things that make it slicker and less stressful for everyone. I am not talking about big things, but just little things that can make a big difference and that is how you learn; you pick up tips from your colleagues and see which ones work for you. It's a personal style thing that makes the difference.

370

COSMO BECOMES A FATHER (DECEMBER 2013)

I asked you before, when you hadn't had much independent experience, whether there was a sense of trepidation in putting someone to sleep - even the colloquialism, 'putting them under', conveys so much power and mystery.

When I am working with a colleague I definitely feel less stress and when on my own it is slowly becoming less stressful. I feel technically confident in most of the individual skills that I need. I don't feel worried that I will do something wrong but it's more about having someone else there who has got the overall plan and responsibility. At the very beginning a registrar might say, 'You are going to learn to do this bit of it,' and they would teach you to put in a line but the rest of it you don't even have to think about.

The next stage is when a senior colleague will explain the plan to you but using the pronoun 'we': 'We are going to use this technique for putting them to sleep and we are going to wake them up in this way.' You are then responsible only for carrying out the instructions and finally somebody comes along and asks you, 'What is your plan for preventing the patient from being sick?' which they may or may not like, because everyone has their own little ways. Now, I've reached the stage when somebody senior will ask me what my plan is and then I go ahead and do it while they may wander off to the coffee room, or assist in another theatre. That's how far I've come, but even though I am now technically executing the plan, if it all were to go wrong, it would still be partly my senior's problem. Whereas, sometimes in those emergencies that happen out-of-hours, I will be all on my own and make and execute my own plan, which I like but it is definitely far more stressful when there is nobody else there to share the responsibility.

And do you see yourself doing this work for the next 35 or more years?

I think so. I remember something I was going to tell you. There are a lot of comparisons drawn between pilots and anaesthetists with the airline industry and its safety records and training. The industry does a lot of simulation and crew resource management, which is all about how failures can be learnt from and flagged up. How you can avoid chains of errors which lead to disaster, which is a big research area in aviation and why aviation is now so safe. Medicine, or primarily anaesthesia, for the last 20 to 30 years, has been trying to learn from the airline industry as to how we can prevent failure. How we learn from near misses, and how you make teams function in a safe way. There is this whole thing in anaesthesia, I don't know how to describe it, but when you do exams, or when you go on courses you are always instructed that if you are in any doubt to go for help. Or, if you are in any doubt then take the safest approach, which may not be the quickest approach, or when in doubt stop, and go back a step. If you are ever unsure, you are taught to do something that may be more difficult, or it may mean the anaesthetic takes longer but it will also be safer. That is how we are trained. However that is not how anaesthesia is always practised.

To go back to the analogy of the pilot – what would a pilot do if the warning light came on before take off? Well, we know he would be expected to turn off all the engines immediately, inform ground-control tower, and to call in a mechanic. In reality that may not always happen, in reality the pilot might say, 'That warning light always comes on, but I've been flying this plane for 30 years and it always goes off again and if we are late we will get a big penalty.' The same thing might happen in anaesthesia.

COSMO BECOMES A FATHER (DECEMBER 2013)

But that goes in the face of what you've just been saying about doubt.

Exactly, but I will tell you. If I saw a patient, it's interesting, if I saw a patient and I thought…how to say this, well, there are a few different ways of keeping someone safe while they are asleep. You can choose to do something that is more invasive, which is to put a tube all the way down into the windpipe. If I do that then their breathing is really, really safe because I have a solid tube all the way down from my machine into the windpipe, directly into the lungs. Or I can put something into the back of their mouth, that goes behind the tongue, which they can breathe through, which is less invasive but not as reliable. You can have problems with something that is less reliable but it is also less invasive, and the patient won't wake up with a sore throat. You don't have to paralyze them while they are asleep and, crucially, they can go home quicker, so there are many advantages. Quite often, if I go to see a patient and then I go to see my boss and I report to him about the patient, 'They have a history of mild asthma and they said they felt sick this morning but they haven't had anything to eat.' I go on to tell him that I would put a tube all the way down, but the response I get back is, 'No need to do that, they will be fine. You don't need to do that.' But, the textbook thing would be, 'Any doubt…'

So, despite the warnings, corners will still get cut?

Yes, and I am aware of that but maybe it is just another reality of life that corners will get cut when maybe people shouldn't cut corners, or maybe they should, I just don't know. I'm not experienced enough. The interesting cultural thing that I've learnt about anaesthesia is you are taught one thing on paper but the undertone, or sub-text, often pushes you in another direction.

I find it both shocking and interesting the preposition 'under' the undertone, comes up again. I anticipate that you would rather have a tube inserted all the way down if you were going under…

Well, not necessarily because there can be complications from it.

Having become an anaesthetist has it now changed your view about submitting to one?

No, not at all but it's not a rational fear, because it is not dangerous but I still don't like the idea of having one. It is that loss of control that's horrible about it. I can see why no one ever wants to have one and why Caroline panicked when she saw that she was to be anaesthetized by someone who was a parallel student to her, even though a postgraduate one.

Except that, once we have lost control, or consciousness, we won't even know that it's happened. And my own experience has taught me that reassurance makes a huge difference. I remember my last words as I went under, and I refused a pre-med precisely because I wanted to stay in control for as long as possible, was telling the surgeon that I was thinking about my beautiful puppy running along a lane. I never got to the end of that lane.

Well, that's true and that's how I look at it too. I once went through a phase of being afraid of flying but now I've taught myself to let go. I tell myself that there is no point being nervous because if we start plummeting towards the ground there is nothing at all that I can do, so enjoy the ride, which I suppose is how I would have to deal with having an anaesthetic.

COSMO BECOMES A FATHER (DECEMBER 2013)

It is essentially about letting go, isn't it?

Yes, that is the only way to deal with it.

I've come to the rather retarded conclusion that applies to a great deal of life. In my profession one can spend a great deal of time exhuming the past but essentially we equally need to learn to teach ourselves, and our clients, how to let go and free fall. Very difficult to 'teach'.

Yes, fears of things you cannot control exhaust you. You finally just have to deal with it. I think that it is a female thing to worry about things that haven't yet happened.

What!

Maybe it's not a female thing. I don't know. I don't know, but I am definitely not scared of things that haven't happened. Then again, some people get nervous about failing exams, and the anxiety can stop them doing well. Am I anxious about Thea getting meningitis? No, I'm not sitting here at all nervous that it could happen, but I am not nervous about it because I have no control over it. With exams I can at least prepare to the best of my ability. One of my ways of dealing with my fears about illness, which includes the fact that at some stage in my life I will need a kidney transplant, and which is a bit annoying but the issue won't go away. The thing that always stops me feeling sorry for myself is that I had a good friend who was at school with me as a kid. It was just a normal day for him, going home from work on his scooter, when he was hit by a taxi and killed. Someone is always going to have it worse than me. And then there's my brother Ben, he's got it worse than me; he is on the list now waiting for a kidney and pancreas transplant. They are not at all easy to perform although the success rate is improving. The other good thing is that you are often transplanted with much younger kidneys because the pancreas must come from a younger person, so you do get quite a good transplant.

What has it felt like seeing your dad go from being one of the most energetic people you could meet, to becoming someone struggling to find the energy for a full week's work?

He is still energetic. I think that he is close to being back to his normal self now. He still overtires himself but it might be good if he starts to reflect on the work life balance. [Silently, I cannot agree with Cosmo about Martin, and I am also thinking how blithely unaware he is that – like two peas in a pod – he might also be talking about himself.] It was very stressful at the beginning when he felt and looked so unwell and we didn't know what the diagnosis was. It could have been 10 times worse, yes much, much worse. It could have been a highly fatal diagnosis. Yes, I offered to go with Dad to the consultation with Dr Glynne to make sure he told me the whole truth. Thinking about my friend who died, which has had a huge impact on me, has reminded me that I didn't tell you about the other very ill child I mentioned that I have looked after.

I was doing one of my first night shifts after I moved to my current hospital, and was called to the Emergency Department by a pager for a 'paediatric cardiac arrest'. On the way to that shift I had been thinking that it would all be fine as long as I didn't have any very sick children to look after, as I still didn't have any formal paediatric anaesthetic experience. I remember hoping that this cardiac arrest call would turn out to be a false alarm but I also

COSMO BECOMES A FATHER (DECEMBER 2013)

knew that a more senior anaesthetist would be coming to assist me, as we work in pairs on 'nights'. We arrived at the same time to find a nine-year-old girl with dark blue mottled skin, in cardiac arrest from severe asthma. There was a team of Emergency Department doctors giving some treatment but with a dire need for help, leadership and some skilled anaesthetic support.

To be honest, Jane, I surprised myself at how decisively I intervened and acted. I was well aware of the theory of the condition and how it should be managed, but I had never seen such a sick child. My senior supported me and allowed me to manage the child all night while we stabilized her and arranged for her transfer to a hospital with Paediatric Intensive Care. It was very stressful and I find myself still often thinking about it, even though I heard that she recovered. It is the only time in my medical career that I feel I stepped in, made a difference and possibly saved a life but I don't know how I would have felt if she had died. It has made me think that in the future I may want to specialize in Paediatric Anaesthesia; I seemed to respond well to the stressful situation and found great satisfaction in it. I was taken by surprise that I have been thinking about this in relation to my future as I have never thought about a career in Paediatrics before.

Loveliest Cosmo, all things change; everything is always invisibly changing before our eyes. When we first met you were the 'child' of our book and now you are both father to little Thea, and becoming the internal father of yourself. It has always struck me that anyone who wants to work with children, and particularly sick children also needs to know how to play...

On the seashore of endless worlds is the great meeting of children.
Rabindranath Tagore

EPILOGUE

The healthy know not of their health, but only the sick: this is the Physician's Aphorism.

Thomas Carlyle

A revolution has occurred in the practice of medicine in the UK. Almost every one of our contributors – regardless of whether they are working in the NHS or have moved into private practice –regret that the changes in a succession of governmental policies have sequestered doctors in the NHS into the counting house where, if they are not partners in a general practice who are accounting to the government for their pennies, they will still be forced to count the minutes they are permitted to spend in patient contact. Aided and abetted by these political changes, our doctors are no longer required to be available out-of-hours for those critical and inconvenient moments when their patients fall ill in the middle of the night, or on a bank holiday. Their 'duty of care' will end with the appointment of a locum. Cosmo has further elucidated this when he protests that he does not want to become a consultant in A&E because he would, in too many instances, not be providing the emergency medicine for which he is trained, but out-of-hours care for the viruses, minor burns and dangerously high night-fevers in infants that GPs used to regard as their vocation to attend. The PC policy of no longer referring to 'patients' (the Latin origin of the word means 'one who suffers'), in bureaucratic favour of the revisionist term, 'service users', speaks for itself.

Patients do not primarily focus on prettier waiting rooms, smiling office staff, or regular newsletters. Rather, they are worried about issues of clinical significance and need to be able to trust the continuity, competence and consistent efficiency of their doctors. They may hold a different view of what is in their best interest from

379

the opinions held by the Department of Health, the Care Quality Commission, NICE or indeed, the Royal College of General Practitioners. Patients know they are in good and competent hands when the care they receive is effectively coordinated, and when they are supported by continuity of care, and health professionals that are well-informed of their individual needs, *histories* and circumstances. The time has come for political action and for a sea-change in the ways in which Primary Care is organized. Forget rewards for doctors who reach targets set by people who do not know or understand the job. Let us now see incentives for doctors who care for their own patients and families and who personally know their histories.

In trying to understand and answer whether there is anything special and unique about doctors and their career choices we want to articulate some of the reasons, both conscious and unconscious, that can act as triggers. Martin and several of our contributors have identified a collective desire that often originates with a childhood fascination in the composition of a dead 'thing'. The desire to know what is going on *inside* of the body, which develops into a subsequent intellectual interest in biology and dissection is at the foundation of medicine and life.

We are reminded of another childhood activity, the archetypal game of 'doctors and nurses', in which almost all children find a socially acceptable channel for their curiosity to explore the biology and pre-pubescent sexuality of childhood. Another unconscious childhood trigger to become a doctor might be the frustration and fear of the child, sometimes as the helpless witness of pain or suffering and premature death in parents, siblings, teachers, or friends. As adults, some of these children may even develop the omnipotent or inflated idea that, by becoming a doctor, they will not only become competent professionals who attend to suffering, but that they will also be able to manipulate and even resort to magical thinking to control their own, and others' health and mortality.

Our contributors have exploded a myth regarding the selection of candidates: the idea that the practice of clinical medicine demands candidates of the highest intellectual rigour. Closer to the truth seems to be an awareness that the study of medicine primarily demands curiosity, memory, the drudgery of repetitive revision, an appetite for constant examinations, which often extend into the candidate's mid-life, and an ability to learn how to jump through hoops. Qualities like sympathy, judgement and a 'healing touch' may only develop after qualification. One further quality that our contributors have identified, and which cannot be taught, but only acquired through fateful intervention, is the concept of 'wounded healer'. Martin, Natasha, Zoe and Rachel have all asserted that doctor becoming patient is a critical *rite de passage* in any doctor's *pharmakon*.

Another observation drawn from these narratives is that every female GP interviewed has acknowledged at least one bout of clinical depression, or a predisposition to hypochondriasis; in stark contrast none of the male GPs have reported a similar episode. A cliché is confirmed whereby the men that we have interviewed claim a greater capacity to compartmentalize and sublimate disillusionment, burnout and depression into work and ambition. Although, when depression does break through in male practitioners, statistics if not these narratives, suggest that the consequences can be more devastating and lead to emotional breakdown, burnout, and even suicide. Not only do the majority of our male doctors favour compartmentalization as a defence against conflict and anxiety, but, with society's disapproval of 'crying men', they may become emotionally and biologically less flexible than women. Women are allowed to signal their distress, fears or even frustration through tears, whereas cultural directives insinuate that it is weak for a man to exhibit lachrymose signs of distress. Taboos against men crying publicly still prevail, which makes it more difficult for them to find a voice with which to signal their distress, or to ask for help.

But a mermaid has no tears and therefore she suffers so much more.
Hans Christian Andersen

It is evident from these narratives that neither male nor female practitioners have escaped from the outrageous slings and arrows, or joys and woes of mortality, which are the emotional price of being born human into a fallen world. The fact that the verb frequently used to signal the onset of illness, 'to fall ill', is a reminder of the myth of the Fall that most poignantly signifies the human condition. Which brings us to express gratitude to all of our contributors, and to thank them not only for their devotion to vocation and for their warrior-like courage, but for the fact that unlike that other great warrior, Coriolanus, who could not bear to remove his linen undergarments, or shield or to display his bloody wounds in the Forum, they have been extravagantly generous in sharing their bruised viscera, inevitable flaws and vulnerabilities with us.

In reflecting back over these stories of life that have been shared, it becomes evident that although every doctor's daily work will bring them face to face with death, our contributors are no more *immune* to death as a result of their training. Perhaps one of the most powerful and unexpected themes running through the book is the impact on several of them of the death of a parent, regardless of whether it was a beloved parent, or one to whom there was primarily a sense of indifference. It is also true that premature death continues to shock everyone and the image of the young mother's dead breast, upon which the nurses had placed a photograph of her newborn baby and a rose, will live on inside most of us.

We are left without doubt, in establishing whether there is anything unique and collectively identifying about the career choice of becoming a doctor, that if society wants to resurrect and preserve the precious and healing tenet of continuity of care, which has been identified as an ideal by so many of our contributors, it is uniquely linked to a sense of vocation. Continuity demands a selfless thoughtfulness and passionate devotion from the doctor to his patients, which is not a professional given, which is immune to inconvenience and which cannot survive in our culture of nine-to-five medicine, and an ad hoc agency provision for out-of-hours contact.

Society hitherto has privileged doctors with an unique authority over our bodies, lives and deaths and in return it has exacted the costly price of devotion, duty and dedication – qualities which now may be in danger of extinction and of becoming anachronisms of medical care and a chimera of one of the most familiar Aristotelian virtues, 'First do no harm.'